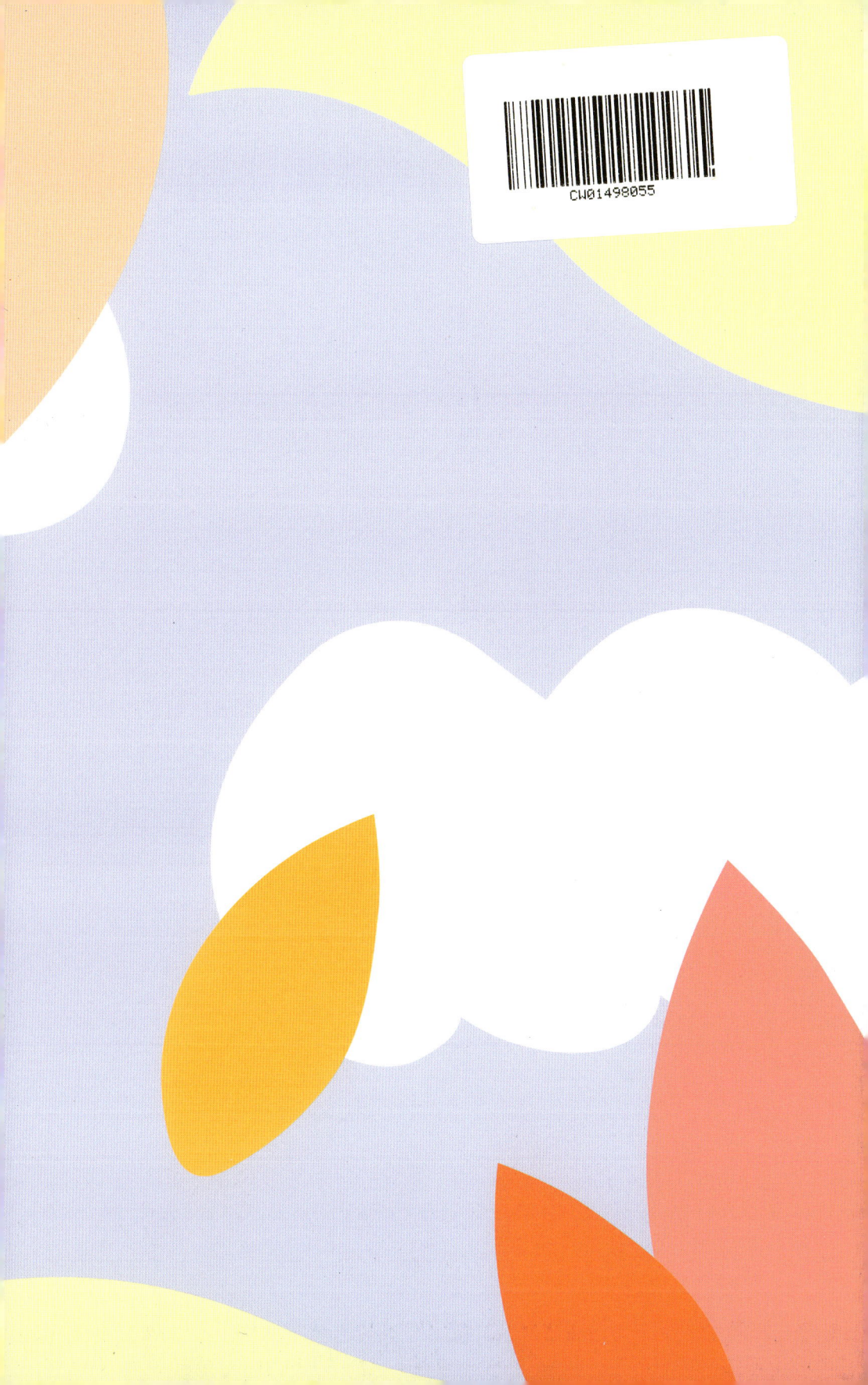

BIRTHING

DAVINA McCALL

WITH MIDWIFE MARLEY HENRY

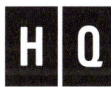

HQ
An imprint of HarperCollins*Publishers* Ltd
1 London Bridge Street
London SE1 9GF

www.harpercollins.co.uk

HarperCollins*Publishers*
Macken House
39/40 Mayor Street Upper
Dublin 1
D01 C9W8
Ireland

10 9 8 7 6 5 4 3 2 1

First published in Great Britain by HQ, an imprint
of HarperCollins*Publishers* Ltd 2025

A catalogue record for this book is available from
the British Library.

ISBN: 978-0-00-870184-0
Special Edition ISBN: 978-0-00-879432-3

Publishing Director: Danielle Pender
Editorial Consultant: Imogen Fortes
Design and Illustrations: Imagist
Senior Production Controller: Halema Begum

While the author of this work has made every
effort to ensure that the information contained in
this book is as accurate and up to date as possible
at the time of publication, medical knowledge is
constantly changing and the application of it to
particular circumstances depends on many
factors. Therefore, it is recommended that
readers always consult a qualified medical
specialist for individual advice. This book should
not be used as an alternative to seeking specialist
medical advice which should be sought before
any action is taken. The author and publishers
cannot be held responsible for any errors and
omissions that may be found in the text, or any
actions that may be taken by a reader as a result
of any reliance on the information contained in
the text which is taken entirely at the reader's
own risk.

With huge thanks to all the brilliant contributors
and wonderful women who shared their stories.

Printed and bound in Italy by Rotolito S.p.A

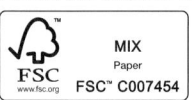

For more information visit:
www.harpercollins.co.uk/green

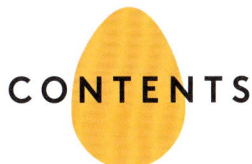

CONTENTS

This book is dedicated to Pam Wilde.

Pam delivered all of our beautiful children. She was responsible for helping me feel totally empowered and full of glorious feminine energy all the way through my births. She died too soon, but I really hope she had some idea of the enormous impact she had on the many babies she brought into this world and the women who gave birth to them ... and their partners too.

Thank you, Pam.
We miss you. 🧡

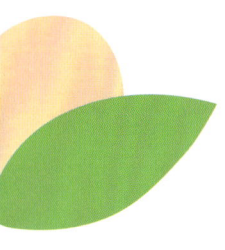

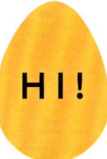

HI!

I want to start by explaining why I'm so passionate about this subject and why I've spent over 24 years wanting to write this book.

It has been 24 years since I first wore the 'BIG MUTHA' T-shirt on *Big Brother* in 2001 and went through the first of three births that I was so lucky to experience. And since having my first baby, I have felt this overwhelming urge to help support and empower women to have the birth they desire and deserve.

Birth, for me, was the most incredible, mind-blowingly amazing experience, but I know it's not like that for everyone. I've heard countless stories from women whose overriding memory of pregnancy and childbirth is fear, anxiety or stress; women who have regrets about their experience, who were let down by their healthcare system, or who simply feel that their birthing process could have been different if they'd been more informed about their options, or they'd had the courage or confidence to speak up when things weren't going the way they wanted. And that breaks my heart. Because while of course certain outcomes are beyond our control, and medical intervention can't alter every childbirth story, I feel so strongly that as a society there are things we can do to support women better through their birthing

journey. And I want to give every woman going forwards the best chance of recounting their birthing stories with the same joy and pride that I, and many other women, do, no matter what direction your birthing story took.

Birthing a baby can be a wonderful, exhilarating rollercoaster of a ride. It can be the hardest thing we ever do as women – squeezing something the size of a football out of our vagina can take us to the limits of our endurance – or it can be a moving experience depending on our circumstances and mindset and I'm going to help you with that later. But it's our ride, our rollercoaster, and we have the **right to decide** how it plays out. There are so many choices to make surrounding birth, and we deserve to have ours respected and adhered to.

Of course, every birth is unique – I've had three children and none of their births was the same. And not every birth will go smoothly or as planned, but I really want to give all of you the best possible chance of having the birth you intended, because too many of us don't or, worse, feel like it was a painful experience we wish to forget.

This book was born (sorry!) out of a desire to change that. I want all of you reading this – as well as your friends, partners and birth supporters – to be able to look back on your birthing journey and feel that you were given every opportunity to have the birth YOU wanted, and to recognise the enormity of what you accomplished. Whether you experience yours in a hospital, at home, by planned caesarean, with an epidural or by conquering the intensity that can at times feel insurmountable, I want to give you the information and the tools you need, to ask for – and receive – the birth you desire. And I want to give anyone supporting you along that path the information *they* need to be the best possible bolster for you.

I want to give you an honest, informative, no-holds-barred guide to birth. As well as sharing my own experiences of being pregnant and giving birth, I'm going to introduce the voices of other incredible lionesses who have brought another human into the world. Throughout the book you're going to read the birth stories of women who've had all different kinds of pregnancy and birthing journeys – the amazing, the heartbreaking, the messy, the moving and the miraculous. They're going to prepare you for the highs – and the lows – and remind you that whatever your experience, you're not alone. Everybody's birth story is unquestionably unique, but somebody somewhere will be able to relate to and understand yours.

As I'm no medical expert, I've worked with the brilliant Marley Henry, a registered midwife and hypnobirthing instructor, who has helped thousands of women give birth, and who has had five babies of her own. I write about the emotional and day-to-day experiences of birth; Marley is going to give you all the practical advice and information, so that together we've armed you with everything you need to know to make your decisions and feel confident in expressing your wishes. I've also assembled an incredible team of other experts who are going to provide specialist advice on topics such as: how to look after your pelvic floor (see page 246); why practising yoga can enhance and support your pregnancy (see page 123); how to support your body via nutrition (see page 66); what to do if you're feeling stressed or have experienced any form of trauma during the birthing process.

Birthing babies didn't just change my life by giving me my children; it gave me a whole new perspective on being a woman, and an appreciation of just how boss, strong, resilient and bloody INCREDIBLE we are. But I've also seen how much shaming there can be around giving birth. I believe the best way to give birth is the way that feels right for you. What matters most is that you come out of it feeling empowered, supported, and proud of what your body and mind have just done.

I described my previous book, *MENOPAUSING*, as a movement and an uprising. *BIRTHING* is my next mission. This book is my way of empowering you to have the birth you desire and deserve. It's my birthing manifesto.

♡ Davina xx

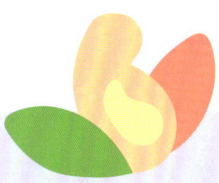

MEET MIDWIFE MARLEY

I've been a registered midwife and hypnobirthing instructor for the past 16 years, both via the NHS and privately. I have supported thousands of women and their families to prepare for parenthood, and cared for them through pregnancy, labour and postnatally. I also have five children of my own, including twins. I am a passionate advocate for empowering women to make informed choices, as to me that is the most powerful tool parents have to try and attain a positive birth experience. Throughout the book, I will be providing practical information and guidance about pregnancy, birth and the postpartum period. This information will be highlighted in purple boxes (as we have here) for ease of use.

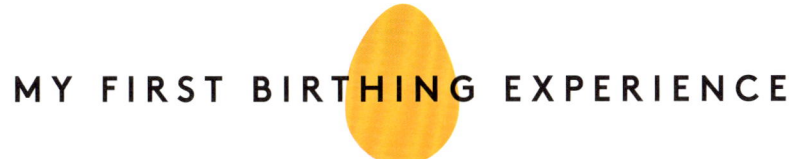

MY FIRST BIRTHING EXPERIENCE

I was 33 when I became pregnant with Holly, my first baby, and to say that I was a slightly anxious new mother would be understating it. We were just about to launch series two of *Big Brother*, and although I'd been on mainstream television for a while, presenting shows like *Don't Try This at Home*, with *Big Brother* I became mega famous almost overnight. I had paparazzi camped outside my house. I'd get tailed everywhere I went. Life became pretty crazy. And that really affected how I started interacting with the world and with other people. I stopped trusting people, because secrets about my life kept coming out in the papers and I didn't understand how (it turned out my phone had been hacked). I was massively in the public eye, and I decided that I wanted to have a baby in a private hospital away from prying eyes and paparazzi. And on that route, I was put in touch with an obstetrician. I was about 16 weeks pregnant, but when I spoke to him, all he could see was problems.

Because what is interesting about seeing an obstetrician when you're pregnant is that generally they are only involved in a birth when there's a problem. Midwives normally guide you through each stage of the process (you will be hearing a load more about what an incredible job they do!), so when I took my scan results to my obstetrician, he started telling me about all the things that could go wrong with my birth and when he would get involved. I left my appointment feeling very nervous. And there's something that happens when you're pregnant and you feel frightened: everything about your pregnancy, which previously felt like the most natural thing in the world, suddenly starts to feel fraught with danger. I went away from that meeting thinking I needed to do some reading of my own because I had to reassure and remind myself that giving birth is a natural process that women have been going through for thousands of years.

Not long afterwards, I was having dinner with some friends. Annabel had just had a baby and she began telling me how much she'd loved giving birth

– that it was the most amazing experience – and I said, 'What do you mean?' She started talking me through her birth, using words like 'empowering' and 'magical', and described her sense of achievement. She'd had her birth at home, and I said, 'You were at home for your first child's birth? Is that not really dangerous?' And she explained that there had been two midwives present and that if they'd sensed any red flags, they would have got her to the hospital, which was nearby, straight away. *This is what I want to hear*, I thought, rather than the doom and gloom of everything that could go wrong. I was about 20 weeks pregnant at that point and asked if I could speak to her midwife, who is an absolute legend called Caroline Flint.

Meeting Caroline changed everything for me. I wasn't one of those football-up-the-jumper types of pregnant woman whom you can't tell are pregnant from behind; I was pregnant in my hands, my feet, my face, my neck – everything just got big. But when I walked in to see Caroline, she said, 'Oh, you look *gorgeous*.' She measured my tummy and said, '*Perfect*.' Every word she used in relation to my pregnancy was positive. She was encouraging and supportive. She put the ball in my court when decisions needed to be made, and when I wasn't sure what my decision would be, she'd leave it with me and say, 'You just let me know when you know.' We talked through the possible options for the birth itself, and I said that I'd quite like to try to give birth at home because that's where I'd feel most relaxed – with all my home comforts around me. I thought I'd feel wrapped up in a nice little cocoon, which was the atmosphere I wanted around me when I brought my baby into the world. I also explained that my husband had reservations about the safety of not being in a hospital.

Caroline told me to talk to my husband and explain that my house was five minutes from a hospital, and that she would call the hospital to let them know when I went into labour, so that they could be ready and prepped if anything were to happen. And from that moment, I never saw the obstetrician again. I just saw Caroline, or Pam, the other midwife who came with her to deliver my daughter Holly.

Giving birth was one of the greatest experiences of my life. I have never felt so proud of myself as I did on each of those three days. I wanted to roar. Pushing a baby out of my vagina felt like the most animal thing I had ever done, and I felt totally in tune with my body. And after I'd given birth, when somebody asked, 'How was it?' I'd say, 'Oh my God, it was f***ing great. I mean, of course, it hurts. You know, you're trying to birth a football, and obviously that's going to be intense, but my God, I loved the ride.' I couldn't wait to do it again. But as I've said, from talking to friends and hearing your stories, it feels as though only about a third or half of us feel like that.

I'm not a home-birth advocate or a natural-birth advocate – that was just my experience, and it was right for me. But there are all kinds of different births that will be affected by time, location and finances. This book isn't about trying to persuade you that any one way to give birth or navigate your pregnancy is right. It's about outlining the options – sharing my story, as well as the experiences and outcomes of other women and men – so that you can make up your own mind about how you want to give birth. So there we have it.

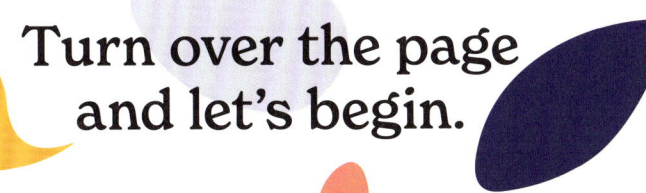

Turn over the page and let's begin.

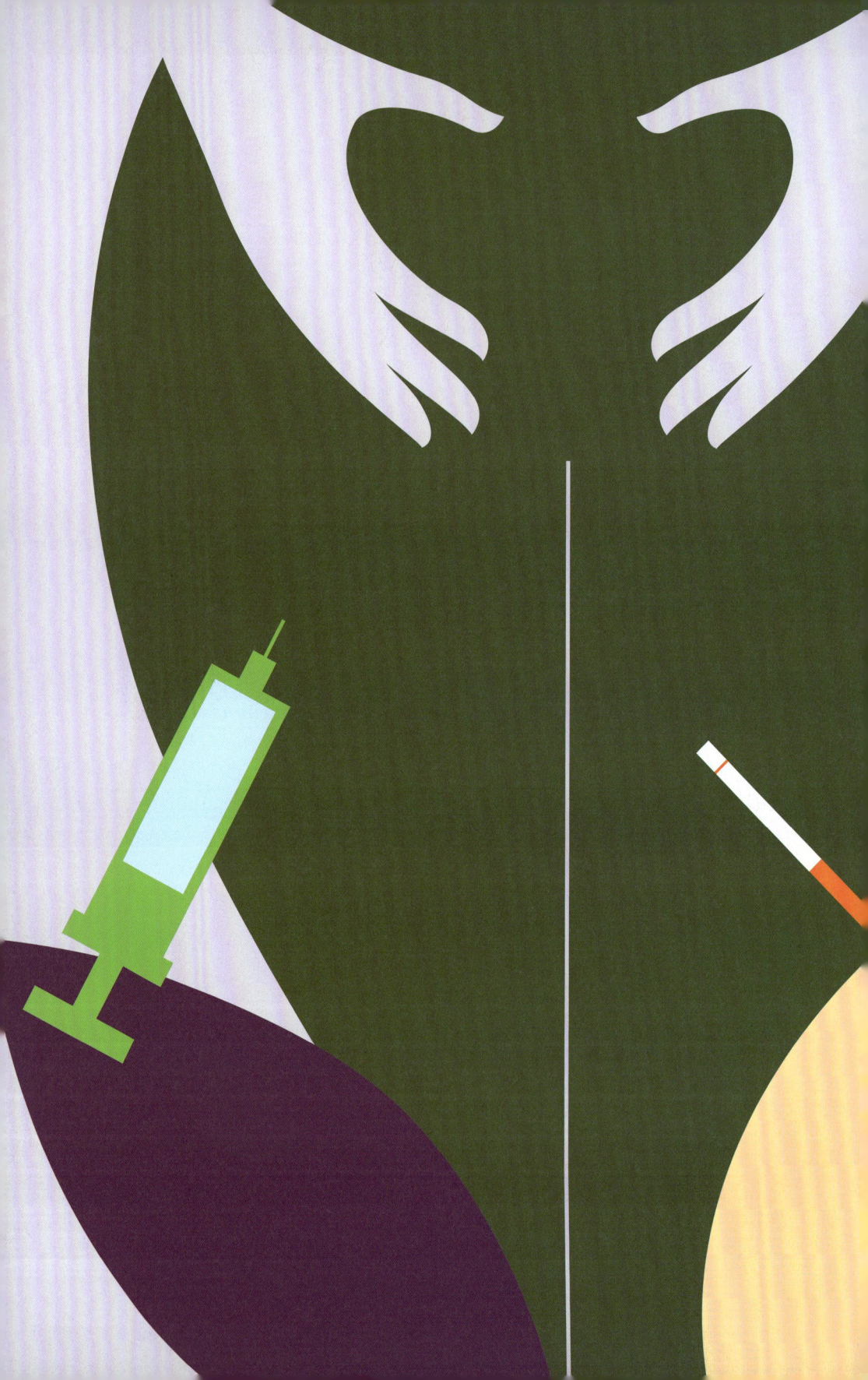

CHAPTER 1

CONCEPTION

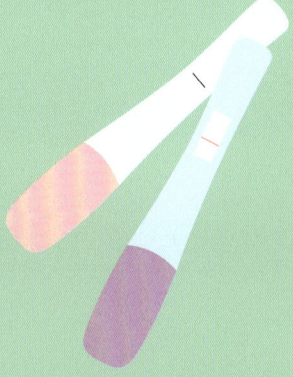

This is the easy part, right?

DECIDING TO HAVE A BABY

I grew up desperate to be a mother. From a really early age I knew that I wanted to look after another person in that way, so by my thirties my biological clock was absolutely screaming at me. But making the decision to have a baby is a very personal one.

Everyone always wants to know, is there a perfect time? And the simple answer is no, so depending on who you are, it's either any time or never. I had such a strong feeling that if I met the right person, and they wanted to have a child, and I felt that we'd make great parents then I would work my life around a baby and I was really lucky that conception happened easily for me and so I was able to plan my career around my pregnancies. But, of course, that's not going to be the case for everyone because it's not usually that simple, and as we'll come to in this chapter, you have to consider the possibility that getting pregnant might not happen easily.

There are so many different reasons a couple or a woman might want to get pregnant, and many factors that will determine when that feels right for them, and the fact is, there is no 'right time' or 'right way' to do it, and no one else's opinion on the subject matters. You might need to think about how taking some time out from your job will affect your career prospects. You might have to consider finances because children can be particularly expensive, or how much support you have around you if that is something that's important to you. If you're a

party animal, you might not want to have a baby because you'll be thinking it will put a stop to all that. But please remember, life is not over because you choose to have children.

For me, one of the most important questions to ask if you're doing this with another person, is are they a good person to raise a child with? Having a baby is hard work and you want to know that this person is going to share the load and the responsibility. How is your relationship going to handle that? Is it going to withstand it? And if you don't think it is, then they're not the person to have a child with.

And then as women reach their thirties, considering the timing for a baby does, in fact, become pretty important. I have lots of girlfriends who are heading towards their late thirties, they would really like to have a family, and some of them are having to think about freezing eggs or realising how hard it is to conceive at this age. And I can see the huge stress that's attached to that and how hard it is for them. So, if having a child is something that you would like to do, then it truly is one of the greatest gifts the universe can bestow on you. I know sometimes it's really difficult to get pregnant. I know time works against you. But if you are with a good person and you want to have one, and they're keen, my advice is just to go for it. There is never going to be a perfect time, so don't waste time and then regret not being able to become a parent.

WHAT HAPPENS WHEN YOU START TRYING

I think there's quite a common belief, especially when we're in our twenties or thirties and we're perhaps one of the first in our friendship group to try to get pregnant, that we make the decision to try for a baby and within a few weeks or a couple of months – wham bam! – that little blue line on the pregnancy test glows and we can settle down and relax because part one is complete.

For many women that is the case, particularly if you're at the younger end of that bracket, but the reality is that for friends I speak to, and so many other women and couples now, it's a completely different story. For them, trying to get pregnant has been months or years of stress and sadness, heartbreak and longing. Many of us are choosing to have children later than our parents or grandparents, and listening to women's stories of assisted reproductive treatment, miscarriage or surrogacy, I know how incredibly lucky I was to have been able to fall pregnant.

When I was thinking about trying to conceive, I was 32. I wasn't aware of anything in my family history that suggested I'd have problems getting pregnant or carrying a baby, but my mum had suffered from ovarian cancer and had to have a full hysterectomy at 28, so I thought it would be a good idea to get everything checked out: to make sure I was ovulating okay and that there weren't any other problems with my fertility.

My fertility test revealed that I had hypothyroidism – an underactive thyroid – which meant that I needed to be put on the thyroid hormone thyroxin. If you have low thyroxine levels it can affect your chances of conceiving, so the blood test was such a useful undertaking for me; it helped me to have the best chance of conceiving.

I got pregnant soon afterwards, but I need to make it really clear from the get-go that making a baby can be really hard. It can take months and months of trying, and there are potential hurdles along the way, which means that some of this chapter is devoted to overcoming the possible obstacles and setbacks.

If you are deciding to start trying for a baby with a partner, it can be a fun time, but it can also turn into a bit of a nightmare time. It starts off being lovely because when you love someone and you're trying for a baby, sex – which was previously something you would do for pleasure alone – becomes something you are doing for pleasure and the possibility of conceiving a life. I think it kind of supersizes the meaning of sex, making it really intense and beautiful. I remember thinking: *Did that make a baby?* But what can also happen is that you try and try and try, and it doesn't work – and it might not work for months, which quickly changes the narrative around sex.

In many ways the stats are really positive: more than 8 in 10 couples, where the woman is under 40, will conceive within a year of having regular unprotected sex (defined as sex every two to three days).[1] And if you've been on the pill and decided to come off it to start trying, once your period returns, there's a high possibility of pregnancy within 12 months. Eighty-three per cent of people who discontinued the pill became pregnant within that time.[2] Keep that stat – 83 per cent is huge.

Despite that, I know many women who are so desperate to get pregnant that if it doesn't happen within the first or second month of trying, they start to feel depressed and deflated. Those feelings can lead to behaviours that make sex and the whole baby-making process not so fun for either person. Lots of women start using fertility trackers and become hyper-aware of the days of the month when they're most fertile, which means they might get a bit tired of just having sex casually and start forcing their partner to get frisky on certain nights. Or they might get angry with their partner if, for example, they've got to go on a business trip during one of their windows for getting pregnant.

'Everyone seemed to be having babies all around me – it was awful.' — Ellen

YOUR STORIES

We started 'trying' for a baby as soon as we got married (not trying before) – and it took two years! Baby number two took even longer (we have a five-year gap) and we eventually had to have IUI treatment (intrauterine insemination) because my body was killing the sperm. The process to get there was painful. Counting, ovulation kits, taking my temperature every day etc. It wasn't enjoyable. Everyone seemed to be having babies all around me – it was awful. IUI worked first time for us. The IUI process was more difficult for my husband,

I believe – it was not all about the woman. But he kept a sense of humour when his sperm came back pink after being washed – 'it wasn't that colour before,' he said. Some family members thought we were meddling but we had a healthy baby.

Davina: I'm so happy you were successful in the end, Ellen. It's so easy to blame ourselves for the setbacks, so thank you for reminding us that it's all about the alchemy between two people, and for sharing your story.

UNDERSTANDING YOUR CYCLE (AND WHEN YOU'RE MOST LIKELY TO GET PREGNANT)

Your menstrual cycle isn't just about your period – it's a complex interplay of hormones that takes place over about a month (usually around 28 days, but it can be a bit shorter or longer – all normal). It's your body getting ready for the possibility of pregnancy, with different phases each playing an important part in this process.

Day 1: the first day of your period, and for most people, bleeding lasts around 3–7 days. After that, your oestrogen levels start to rise and your body starts prepping to release an egg. You might feel a bit more energetic and more up for it (yep, that's the hormones too).

Day 14 (ish): ovulation – the main event. This is when your body releases an egg, and that's your fertile window – the few days when you're most likely to get pregnant. Sperm can hang around in your body for up to seven days, so if you're trying to conceive, having sex in the days leading up to and just after ovulation gives you the best chance.

After ovulation, progesterone rises, which can make you feel a bit more sluggish, more hungry, or emotional; and if the egg isn't fertilised, your hormone levels drop and your period arrives again.

The key thing? Every woman's cycle is slightly different, and it might take a couple of months of tracking to understand your rhythm. Whether you're using apps, ovulation tests or just paying attention to how you feel, tracking it can be an important part of your conception journey.

Every woman's cycle is slightly different, and it might take a couple of months of tracking to understand your rhythm.

KEEPING TRACK OF YOUR CYCLE

Timing is everything when you're trying to conceive, so understanding your cycle and being able to track and predict your fertile window is vital for success. Happily, there's been a massive rise in 'femtech' (female technology, for any other technophobes like me out there) over the past decade, which is designed to help you understand and exploit your windows of opportunity. There are loads of fertility apps available now; the ones below are some of those that have been recommended to me and are easy to use (most are free but premium features may require a subscription):

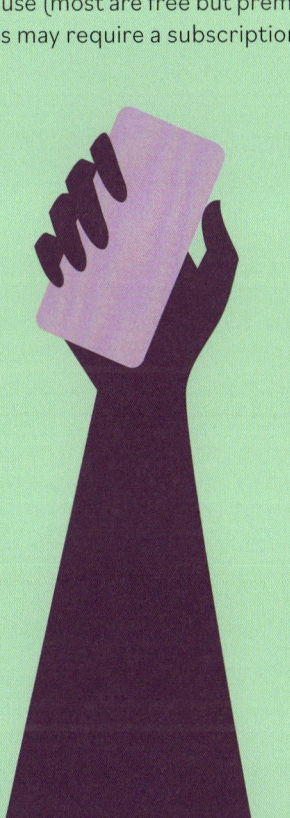

— **FLO** claims to be the world's most popular female health app. Once you input your period dates, it will be able to give you an idea of how long your cycles are and tell you which week you're most fertile – it even gives you an idea of the exact ovulation date. You can also input results from ovulation tests if you're using them, plus there is a pregnancy mode to help track your baby's development and remind you of any appointments.

— **Kindara** is one of the more sophisticated apps; it helps you to understand your body and your reproductive health, and makes predictions based on your data. It offers a vaginal sensor that captures your core basal body temperature wirelessly and can record data, such as your cervical mucus, when you've had sex.

— **Clue** helps you predict your menstrual cycle by tracking over 100 experiences connected to your cycle, such as feelings, cravings, PMS, sex drive and more. Like Flo, you can also use it to track your baby's development.

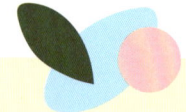

TRYING FROM A POET'S PERSPECTIVE

Harry Baker, Poet

My experience of male friends trying for a baby was them tentatively mentioning it as a New Year's resolution and then following it up a few months later with a joyful announcement. When the time came for us to start trying, I was looking forward to doing the same.

The first few months genuinely felt like an extra reason to have sex, followed by a nervous excitement when my partner's period was due. By six months in, I noticed a sadness had crept into these monthly revelations, but I reasoned that it was her body and not mine, so I didn't have a right to be more upset than she was. By the time it got to a year, it felt like we had been foolish to leave it so long to start trying and expect it to happen immediately. At two years in, we started to make enquiries with the GP just in case.

Part of what made it so hard was that there was no obvious moment of pain or grief to share with others, just an increasing heaviness as the months rolled on. Some days would be absolutely fine, and some days, I would feel an aching loss for a life that hadn't even happened yet.

I didn't know how to bring it up with friends who I had mentioned it to at the start of the year, even though it was obvious that no joyful announcement had followed. Me and my partner made sure to check in with each other, and she often seemed more stoic than I was. In part because she had spoken to friends who had gone through miscarriages and IVF and therefore knew that it wasn't straightforward, whereas I had never had those conversations, even though I was often just as good friends with the men in those relationships.

It was around this point that I started to write my poem 'Trying'. In the process of attempting to articulate what had been such an isolating experience, I was finally able to open up to other male friends, too (even if that started by pulling out of a cycling holiday because I wanted to protect my testicles). I was astonished at how similar some of their experiences had been and felt awful that I hadn't been there for them in the same way.

It gave a language and an excuse for being able to check in, whether it was the friends making sure their own pregnancy announcement wouldn't upset us or the mate telling me they were there if I ever needed to talk about 'the thrills and spills of wanking into a cup'.

When I started to read the poem at gigs, I knew how powerful it was to be able to share what I was going through, and I was moved by how many people had seen their own stories reflected as well. I'm honoured that Davina has asked me to share the poem here, and I hope it encourages people (especially men) to talk about their own experiences further because that made all the difference for me.

TRYING

Harry Baker, Poet

I have this friend who is
trying to have a baby.
Although *trying* might not
quite be the right word.
As their partner put it,
they were no longer trying
not to have a baby.

Which becomes
not wanting to plan anything more than
nine months in advance, just in case.
Becomes making the most of this
Christmas or summer as a two, because
soon everything's going to change.
Becomes two parallel realities
coexisting the moment a period's late.
Becomes focusing on doing
the things they can no longer do
when they do have a baby.
Becomes if they do have a baby.

And it is trying. And they are trying.
But *trying* suggests
they could be trying harder.

Suggests they are not
trying hard enough.
Suggests they are trying and failing.

At some point trying becomes aching.
Becomes longing. Becomes praying.
And in some ways it is
the ultimate act of faith.

Maybe *hope* is the best word – it often is.
Because hope still comes with doubt.
I'm just hoping that
their hope doesn't run out.

You see, my friend is hoping to have a baby.
Although *have* perhaps
isn't quite the right word.

In German, one of my
favourite verbs is *machen*.
It means to carry out, to make, or to do.

In English, you *take* a photo.
In German, you *make* a photo.
In English, you *go on* holiday.
In German, you *make* a holiday.
In English you *have* indecision.
In German, you don't.

In English you *have* fun.
In German you *make* fun.
It feels less concerned with ownership
and more with creativity.
As I think we all should be.

What I'm saying is my friend
isn't hoping to take or have a baby.

But I think they'd really like
to make or machen ein baby.

I have this friend who is
hoping to make a baby.
Although *friend*, it tends to
not be the right word.

More like friends.

There is the friend who told me
four years ago that they thought
that now might be their time.
And then they hadn't mentioned it since,
so I figured that maybe
they'd just changed their mind.

The friend whose partner isn't against it
but wants to wait before thinking of kids.
And yet her body is different to his,
so she is not sure she can
live with that risk.

The friend who would be
such a brilliant mum,
according to everybody that they know.
They just thought that they
would have a partner by now,
and they don't want to do this alone.

The friends who both
wanted kids for a while,
and both committed to try IVF,
but had to spend £25k privately
before they could apply to the NHS.

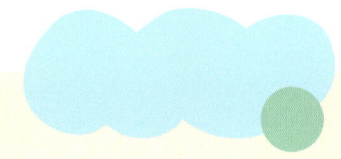

Because they are both women.
And that is the only way to prove
that they are trying.
But they are trying.
They are all trying. And aching.
And longing. And praying.

I have these friends
who are hoping to make a baby.
Although *baby* maybe
isn't the right word.
Because most of my friends
that do have babies are exhausted.
And having friends
that do have babies is ideal,
because you get to have a cuddle
and then give them back.

And anyway, surely
the best bit's the next bit.
Because you are not just
making a baby, but a child.
And they have not only
learnt to walk and talk,
but to run down the street
chanting your name,
and if you do anything they think is funny,
they will ask you to do it again.
And again. Forever.

And in any given situation,
they would rather play than chat.
And I will be honest: I am thirty-one,
and I still feel like that.
When they are at that age
they do not *have* fun; they *make* fun.

And while you cannot
possibly know how it turns out.

When they value creativity over ownership,
or attempt to run a marathon
every now and then,
you will know some of that is down to you,
and you will make sure they know
you are so proud of them.
Because you are not just making a baby,
or a child, but a life.

I have these friends who are
hoping to make a life.
And so am I.

And yet, out of all of the friends
that I mentioned,
almost all talked about it in passing,
and only one of those friends is a guy.
And I have messaged about since, asking.
And for whatever reason he doesn't reply.
But I am trying.

I am trying to talk about it.
I am trying to hold it lightly.
I am trying to not get my hopes up.
But I like getting my hopes up.

When I hear somebody say
they are expecting a baby
I realise that is exactly what I have
been doing for years now.

When anyone asks me if I have kids
I say I have three incredible nieces.

And three amazing godsons.
Or that having friends with babies is ideal
because you get to have a cuddle
and then give them back.
But one day I would love to be the one
you give them back to.

And I am so grateful to the friends
who knew what we were going through,
and so were sensitive to us
when sharing their incredible news.
Especially the friend who, four years ago,
said they thought now was their time,
because now is their time.
Even if it means that when I message
he takes a while to reply.

But the best is the friend
with a one-year-old,
who she obviously loves to bits,
and yet she says she spends
so much time wondering
what her life would be like without kids.
How it must be nice. And it is.

My partner says the hardest part
is the not knowing.
Being stuck in the in-between
of now and might-never-come-to-be.
The truth is right here. Right now.
I know that my life doesn't feel incomplete.
And, whichever reality that we end up in,
I am so grateful that she is with me.

And I still think I'd be a good dad.
But I guess there's no way to know.
At least I have made a head start
on the list of things that I cannot control.

While I cannot possibly know
how it turns out,

I have these friends.
And I have hope.
And I am already making a life.

Or at least
I am trying.

To watch Harry perform his
absolutely incredible poem,
'Trying', scan this QR code.
I can't recommend it
highly enough.

YOUR STORIES

'We tried for a few years to conceive with no luck. Whenever we met couples who fell pregnant we'd smile politely but inside it ate us up.' — Kazimierz

I was working a stressful job and felt it was a me issue, which as a man can be incredibly painful. Low and behold I quit the stressful job and we fell pregnant almost straight away.

Then it came to the birth prep. Only after doing a few birth courses did I realise quite how important a role I had. It wasn't just that so long as the baby is alright nothing else matters, my wife wanted to feel empowered and the whole system of giving birth is designed to take that away. I found myself (politely) batting away medical interventions on her behalf while also judging what was the right call. Because of the prep my wife made us do, I didn't feel like a lemon, I was able to be helpful.

We both came out of the experience content that we'd got the best birth(s) we could but it was only because we really knew what she wanted.

Davina: Kazimierz, thank you so much for sharing this. It's really important to have men's perspectives in this book, and to understand how hard it is from your side when there are problems getting pregnant. But the fact that you are here, thanking your wife for coming on this journey with you, and that both of you were super prepared and knew what you wanted is just so lovely to hear. Thanks so much for telling us your story.

SEX AND CONCEIVING

If you are trying to get pregnant with a partner, I would recommend that you don't tell them when you are fertile. It's fine for you to know; you can do all the ovulation sticks you want. I mean, Jesus, I spent a small fortune on pee sticks to find out if I was ovulating or not. Just don't tell your partner, because if you do, suddenly sex and intimacy can start to feel fake – more like work – because you are doing them purely to make a baby. And after a while, if it's going on for a long time, that can really start to take its toll on your sexual relationship and on how you interact with your partner.

So, we've asked the wonderful Dr Karen Gurney to talk about how to navigate this experience and make sure you get through it with honesty and openness so that you're still having great, healthy sex, as well as trying to conceive.

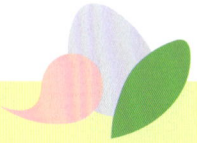

CONCEPTION, STRUGGLES TO CONCEIVE AND YOUR RELATIONSHIP

Dr Karen Gurney, Consultant Clinical Psychologist

For some people, the period of time leading up to a positive pregnancy test might have been heavily focused on struggling to conceive. Sex might have become boring, predictable, associated with stress rather than desire, and something that, once you got pregnant, you felt quite happy to take a bit of a break from. Feeling like this after trying to conceive is totally normal. It's also likely to affect one or both of you for some time post-birth. Is this something you've ever talked about with your partner? Many people can be quite ashamed of these feelings, as they seem to take the shine off the romanticism around conception, or they worry that it says something about their sexual relationship. The truth is, these are normal feelings to have, and acknowledging them can allow you to open up a conversation about needing to do things differently for a while.

You have a couple of options to redress the impact of trying to conceive. Firstly, it's okay to have some time off. In fact, one of the best things you can do is forget about sex for a bit and focus on the sexual currency between you. (This is a term I coined to describe the sexual charge between you and a partner, outside of sex acts. For example, flirting, passionate kissing, suggestive texts, saying, 'You look hot today.' Sexual currency is part of our sex life and can decline the longer we have been together. It can help us feel sexually connected even when sex feels out of reach. This is very helpful for parents!) Another change that will help is to enjoy finally taking the focus away from penis-in-vagina sex and having a bit more variety in your sex life – for example, sex sessions that are just kissing passionately for 15 minutes, one of you giving the other oral sex, or making each other come with your hands. All of this **is sex** and can often be much hotter than the type of sex you had in a formulaic way when trying to get pregnant. Changing up your sex life after trying to conceive can bring with it a novelty-induced spike in desire that allows you both to reset. Societal expectations about what sex

looks like (i.e. 'sexual scripts' of who does what and when, and restrictive ideas of what constitutes 'real sex') can make it hard to do this without open discussion, hence the need to have an honest conversation about the impact of trying to conceive on both of you.

You may find it useful to discuss what you need from each other moving forward. For example, are you nervous to initiate sex because you felt rejected? Do you need more compliments on your appearance to feel sure your partner still finds you attractive? Did you find sex more enjoyable when it was less predictable and want more of this? Did you get so used to not being sexual that you feel you both need to make a real effort to bring your sexuality back together? Do you need a break from sex, or at least a break from penis-in-vagina sex, to bring back some novelty again?

Ideally, share your answers, and make a commitment to use this information for the good of your sex life in future. The real value here is in hearing each other out and going easy on one another. Sometimes challenges around sex can make us feel like we are on different teams, but remember, you are on the same team, and you both need to hear what the other feels and needs.

DESIRE AND DISAPPOINTMENT

The other thing I would add to this is try to be subtle at sexy time, because if you are suddenly bringing out the belly-dancing costume or getting the Ann Summers gear on when you've never worn anything like that before, you may unconsciously be creating unrealistic expectations in your partner, as you may not be able to sustain that kind of sexiness for them in the long term (it may also inspire you to take this kind of frisky behaviour forwards!). And then, once you've stopped trying for a baby, it would be understandable for your partner to mourn the loss of this desperately horny person and colourful sex life (or it may be the beginning of a whole new era in your sex life!). What I'm saying is, it's a sensitive time.

Conception can be one of the most fun, exciting parts of your relationship, but if it starts getting desperate, that quickly goes south. If you need to offload to somebody about ovulating and being fertile, talk to your friends, not your partner. So, as hard as it is – and I do know how difficult it is not to get a bit desperate about conceiving; I was that person – try to remember that 83 per cent of people get pregnant within a year, which makes anything up to a year normal. This is important because, as I will come back to quite a lot over the course of this book, stress is really bad for the body and is an enemy of conception. If after a year you are struggling to conceive and your fertility test hasn't flagged anything to worry about, you could talk to your GP about going to see a fertility expert.

YOUR STORIES

'We'd heard it would take a while.' — Zara

So we went into it relaxed. No tracking apps. Just a quiet agreement to stop being careful and see what happened. And then it did. Almost immediately. I remember staring at the test, heart racing. We were thrilled and grateful, of course – but also stunned. We'd imagined a slow build, time to get our heads around the idea, to savour the final stretch of just being us. Instead, everything shifted overnight. We went from wine on a Friday night and weekend lie-ins to reading about folic acid and foetal development. The 'just us' era closed faster than we were ready for. No one tells you how quickly the dynamic

can change. We're still learning how to hold on to each other. Still figuring out how to be us, now that there's about to be three.

Davina: It is so interesting that you look forward to conception and are praying that everything's going to work, that it is easy to forget to think about the impact it might have on your relationship. It is good to talk about this before you conceive, and how you're both going to nurture and care for the relationship once you get pregnant and have a baby. Thank you for flagging this because I think this is really important.

LOOKING AFTER YOUR BODY

I'm obviously going to be the person who tells you that exercise and what you eat should be at the forefront of anything health-related, but they definitely should be on page one of your journey to conception and pregnancy; they are so important. When you're thinking about trying to conceive, what you want to do is try to get your body primed and into shape to give it the best possible chance of being able to house a fertilised egg.

To help you with that preparation I've asked the absolutely incredible registered dietician Dr Federica Amati, who is the head nutritionist at ZOE, to explain how you can support your body through what you eat at this time.

You're going to be hearing lots more from Federica as we go through the book, as she'll be providing advice on what to eat throughout your pregnancy.

'Creating the best possible environment to get pregnant begins roughly 90 days before conception.' — Dr Federica Amati

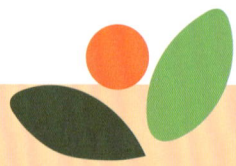

EATING FOR CONCEPTION

Dr Federica Amati, Nutritionist

The first 1,000 days is the most critical period of development in all of the human life course and it starts at conception. Conception is a statistically unlikely and biologically miraculous moment where the right sperm with the right attributes is welcomed by a womb that is ready for pregnancy, reaches an egg ready to be fertilised in its specific 24-hour window and the two successfully combine, blending their genetic information to spark the beginning of a potential new life.

There are dozens of factors that help support our chances of conception. Creating the best possible environment for this to happen begins roughly 90 days before conception, when the immature egg and primordial sperm cell begin their evolution to prepare for their expedition to new life.

Both eggs and sperm can vary hugely in quality; from the sperm's ability to swim – and swim in the right direction – to the sperm's shape and quality of the DNA they carry, to the eggs' ability to select the 'right' match for best possible success of conception. Quality and function are impacted by age, though ageing for eggs has a compound effect because we have all of our eggs from when we were made in our mother's wombs, meaning they are exposed to the elements of our lives from the start. But it is not just how many years you've lived on this planet that makes the difference; your time stamp since birth and genetics can mean something very different depending on how well you have cared for your body in that time. Eating well, moving functionally throughout the day, mitigating the impact of stress and looking after your mental health, and limiting your exposure to harmful chemicals like alcohol, vaping and smoking have a huge role to play in how 'old' your eggs and sperm really are.

The dietary pattern that clearly supports our best chances of conception is the Mediterranean Diet. This is a diet rich in leafy green vegetables, tomatoes, fresh herbs, legumes and beans, whole grains, nuts and seeds, extra virgin olive oil, and fruit as the majority of daily food choices. This means that more than half of your plate should be made up with these whole plants dressed with the best dietary fat we know of – extra virgin olive oil. Adding oily fish, such as salmon, mackerel, anchovies, sardines, mussels and even oysters is an important addition to get beneficial omega-3 fatty acids and zinc in the diet. Eating eggs, natural yoghurt and cheese is a wonderful way to get nutrient density in delicious foods and eating good-quality meat once or twice per week can be part of a healthy diet. Avoid regularly eating processed meats like bacon, industrially made cakes, biscuits, pastries, snacks and ready-meals, opting instead – where possible – to make your own. Drinking alcohol is not good for us and it is especially unhelpful when trying to conceive, so cutting that right down to one occasional drink, or none at all, is the best advice.

If you are trying to conceive, establishing a healthy diet is the best tool to improve fertility and to ensure you have the best nutritional status to support your pregnancy, birth and parenthood. Supplementing should always be discussed with your doctor or nutrition professional (a registered dietitian (RD) or registered nutritionist (RNutr)) as the only supplements that are recommended for those trying to conceive are folic acid, vitamin D,

choline and omega-3 if you do not eat fish. Supplements at any dose do not replace the beneficial impact of a healthy diet and can be harmful in some cases. Being undernourished – i.e. not getting enough nutrients and energy from your food – reduces the chances of conception as we have evolved to avoid conceiving where there isn't enough food available, such as during a famine.

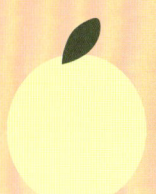

THE IMPACT OF STRESS

I am not an endocrinologist, so I won't attempt to explain the science behind the hormones that trigger stress, and its impact on conception and fertility. But what I can tell you is that there are times when I can really feel that stress is having a negative impact on my body.

In 2017 I presented a fascinating programme called *The Davina Hour*, which looked at the dilemmas and challenges we're facing as a society, and one of them examined stress. It was really interesting, because the effects of stress are so much more wide-reaching than I'd thought. Some of the physical signs include panic attacks, sleep problems, fatigue, muscle aches and headaches, indigestion and heartburn, but stress can also affect your thought processes and how you feel; it can impact your sleep, make you feel anxious and lead to health problems such as high blood pressure, heart disease, stroke, obesity and diabetes.

The bottom line is that when we are trying to conceive, we want to minimise stress as much as possible because studies have shown that while it's unlikely that stress alone can cause infertility, it does interfere with our ability to get pregnant, as does anxiety.

But how do you combat your stress? That's the big question. Here are some of the strategies I recommend:

1 **HAVE A CHAT**

Talking to someone is really helpful. Try to talk through what you're stressed about, because carrying a burden on your own can feel very lonely, frightening and isolating, which can cause more stress. Talk to other people experiencing problems conceiving. Tell friends who you know will empathise. And talk to your partner – communicate with them and make them feel part of this process rather than shutting them out (but as we discussed, read the room and try not to impact your sex life). Be a team and tackle the tough times together.

2 **GET MOVING**

I know I bang on about this, but a little bit of exercise really can help you get through stress and offload it. Exercise is so good for your mental health and is such an effective way to manage stress. Anything – even just a 20-minute walk to get out into nature, feel the wind on your face and take some deep breaths – can be so healing and helps calm your mind.

3 **CHILL OUT**

And I mean really relax. Designate some time for doing something that calms you and makes you feel good, something that allows you to completely switch off. For me, it's having a bath with some music on. Another thing I do to relax is exercise.

I know that sounds weird, but when I'm exercising, especially if I'm following a class online, I genuinely don't think about anything other than what I'm doing. I find it really meditative.

4   HELP OTHERS

It can really help to do something for someone else, as it takes you away from your own problems. Try calling someone else who's going through a challenging time and do your best to help them or just be an ear for them, rather than thinking about your own worries.

5   SAY THANK YOU

Writing out lists of all the things in your life that you're grateful for has been proven to help relieve stress. Expressing gratitude for people, things and events by writing them down can help strengthen your emotional resilience and reduce stress, as you're focusing on all the positives, rather than your problems.[4]

6   MEDITATE

Meditation is quite a difficult one, as lots of people find it hard, but there are different ways you can meditate. The best option if you're struggling with it is to use an app that has guided meditations. I have a monthly subscription to the Headspace app because I've found that 15–20 minutes each day really helps me, but if you don't want to commit to the cost of something like that (Insight Timer and Calm are also both good), there are lots of free resources on YouTube.

7   SHAKE THE ROOM

I know it might sound weird, but shaking – like a dog shakes to dry off and relieve stress – is really brilliant for stress relief. And I've definitely found it a real release. I'm not sure if it is a physical thing, but I promise you, shaking really has helped me – I've also laughed a lot while doing it, which helps get rid of stress. There is actually some evidence to support the idea that shaking can help regulate the nervous system and calm the body when it's overstimulated.[5] The technique isn't rocket science, but if you look up the concept of shaking for stress relief, there are a few good videos on YouTube.

8   BREATHE

I know I'm slightly behind the curve, but I recently went to my first breathing class with a breathwork practitioner, and it absolutely blew my mind. The space you can get yourself into, mentally, just by breathing, is incredible. It's extremely meditative and is an amazing way to feel more empowered in your body and less out of control. I believe breathwork is an invaluable tool that can help everyone cope with the stresses of conception, the enormity of labour and just generally be absolutely life-enhancing. Louise Oliver is a GP, functional breathing practitioner and therapeutic life coach who's brilliant at explaining how to calm yourself by using the breath. If you go to her website (see page 309), you'll find lots of super-helpful advice, and on the next page she's put together tips and practical exercises for avoiding and managing stress to help you navigate this time.

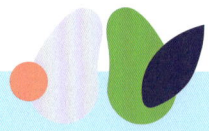

HOW WE BREATHE MATTERS

Dr Louise Oliver, Therapeutic Life Coach

The human body is amazing; it is constantly making adjustments to its unconscious processes, such as breathing, blood pressure, hormone production and sexual organ function, in response to external stimuli. These processes are controlled by our autonomic nervous system (ANS), which is divided into two main parts:

— **Sympathetic nervous system ('fight, flight, freeze' system)**
When activated, the body prioritises the bodily functions required to survive the next few seconds and minutes, such as muscle contraction and releasing sugar, cortisol and adrenaline into the blood.

— **Parasympathetic nervous system ('feed and breed' system)**
When activated, the body prioritises the bodily functions needed for longer-term survival, such as digestion, libido, conception, pregnancy and labour.

Both systems are always active, but the body is constantly adjusting the dial between the two of them. So, how can we consciously control the ANS? One amazing tool is to deliberately alter how we breathe.

Consider over the next week how you breathe throughout the day and night. The body associates breathing quickly and noisily, through an open mouth and using our upper chest, with a threat and therefore turns up the dial on the 'fight, flight, freeze' system when this happens. Breathing slowly and quietly, in and out of the nose, using the diaphragm, helps the body feel safe, which boosts our 'feed and breed' system. Is your breathing sending safe or threatening signals to your body? By working with your breath to turn up the dial on your 'feed and breed' system, you will be boosting your libido, helping you to conceive and become a parent, thereby reducing stress, which is counterproductive if you're trying to conceive.

If your breathing is not already like this, you can change it. The best time to do this is before you start trying for a baby, but you can change it at any time.

Be kind and patient with yourself, as it takes time to change your unconscious breathing pattern by creating new nerve connections and altering muscle memory, but it can be life-altering in so many ways. One helpful way to start is by practising the breathing exercise below.

Other ways to increase the 'feed and breed' system include calming activities such as mindfulness, meditation, spending time in nature, listening to calming music, singing and humming. Reducing stress, human touch, massage, laughter, deliberate cold exposure and practising kindness are also beneficial.

Breathing is generally automatic; however, it is not automatically efficient.

We can breathe efficiently, inefficiently or anywhere in between.

Efficient breathing is breathing slowly, quietly, in and out of the nose, using the diaphragm.

How we breathe during wakefulness influences how we breathe during sleep.

It is important to have a healthy, efficient ANS during pregnancy and labour, given the huge demands placed on it by the bodily changes, and breathing well day and night increases the likelihood of having a healthy, effective ANS.[6] As pregnancy progresses, breathing generally becomes more inefficient due to the increase in fatty tissue, circulating blood volume, water retention and nasal congestion, and the restricted movement of the diaphragm.[7] So improving breathing efficiency before becoming pregnant may help the ANS control bodily functions such as blood pressure, pulse and muscle movement during pregnancy and labour.

Women also have an increased risk of sleep disordered breathing (SDB) during pregnancy, and there are growing concerns that this may increase the risk of complications for mothers and babies during pregnancy, labour and the postpartum period.[8,9,10,11] SDB includes a range of conditions related to breathing difficulties during sleep, such as the airway becoming narrowed or blocked. Individuals may snore, breathe noisily or have gaps in breathing while asleep, often leading to daytime sleepiness and fatigue. Smoking tobacco, recreational drug use and having a higher body mass index (BMI) are all factors associated with SDB in pregnancy,[12] so addressing these factors before you get pregnant can be beneficial. It is advisable to discuss any concerns about SDB before or during pregnancy with a health professional.

Breathing slowly and quietly, in and out of the nose, helps the body feel safe.

How we breathe while moving, resting and sleeping matters. We can change how we breathe.

BREATHING EXERCISES TO ACTIVATE THE 'FEED AND BREED' SYSTEM

You have the power to alter how you breathe to achieve the outcome you desire. These exercises will help you breathe in a way that supports the reproductive process. The tongue, the diaphragm (our main breathing muscle) and the pelvic floor are connected,[13] so the first steps are designed to improve your breathing posture.

— **Step 1:** The correct position for the tongue is against the roof of the mouth with light suction, the tip of the tongue on the ridge behind the front teeth. Your lips should be sealed and your teeth unclenched. Try to train your brain to remember this position unconsciously by practising it whenever you get a drink and go to the toilet.

— **Step 2:** Good posture helps us to breathe as nature intended. Imagine a string gently pulling you up from the back of your head, helping you stand tall. Relax your shoulders, put your tongue in the correct position, as described, and begin to breathe silently in and out of the nose.

— **Step 3:** When this feels comfortable, try breathing more slowly.

— **Step 4:** When you're ready, try making the exhale longer than the inhale. Then, as you inhale, imagine the air moving through the nose and travelling down into the bottom of your lungs, pushing the lower ribs outwards. Feel the relaxation as you allow the breath to naturally leave your body through your nose and as your lower ribs move inwards.

— **Step 5:** After practising this, you might like to try inhaling silently through your nose for four seconds and exhaling silently through your nose for six seconds, while continuing to feel the movement of your lower ribs.

— **Step 6:** Try regularly breathing in this manner, perhaps while watching TV or before bed to help you relax.

Time spent practising this exercise turns up the relaxation response, turns down the fight, flight, freeze response, and develops the flexibility within your ANS to manage the challenges of conception, pregnancy and childbirth. If at any point during these exercises you feel hungry for air or you develop tension while breathing, take a 10–20 second break, then try again. If you are still struggling, I have more information on my website and more specific guidance related to pregnancy: drlouiseolivertherapeutic lifecoaching.com/.

WHAT IF YOU'RE NOT GETTING PREGNANT

When you're having problems conceiving, there are so many things going on in your head. First, you might be feeling like a failure, wondering why everybody around you seems to be able to get pregnant so easily (generally speaking, we're often trying to conceive at the same time as many of our friends and contemporaries) when you can't. You start doubting yourself, your body, your partner. Sometimes, if it's just not happening for you, an obsessive thinking pattern can take over your whole life. You wake up in the morning, you think about it. God forbid, the first day of your period comes; it's devastating. You tell your partner, and they feel sad because you are telling them in a sad way. And that then impacts on you because you feel bad because you can't get pregnant. You might feel like there's something wrong with you. It's a vicious cycle that can be extremely difficult to cope with, and often feelings of jealousy or frustration arise when somebody else announces they're pregnant. This is completely normal. Please don't feel like a bad person. But it makes you question yourself. When this pattern carries on for a while, some people start to feel depressed, anxious or lonely, and above all completely powerless.

Add to this the fact that all of these emotions can trigger stress, which, as we know, is bad for the body,

particularly when you're trying to conceive, and essentially what you have is the perfect storm. Studies confirm that depression levels in patients with infertility are the same as those in patients who have been diagnosed with cancer and heart disease.[14]

So, I really want to encourage you to try to manage your expectations. The time between trying for a baby and then waiting for your period to come is generally around two weeks. Try not to think about it too much during that time. Stay busy. Have some fun. See mates. Do everything you can to minimise your worries and not put too much pressure on yourself. If you're doing this with your partner, keep having sex. Of course, making a baby will still be something you're thinking about, but when you come to do a pregnancy test, try (try!) to keep your expectations measured. I know it's exciting, but that excitement can also trigger massive disappointment if the test is negative. Maybe wait until your period is at least one day late to do the test.

It's also really important to hold on to all the things you love about your partner. If there are things you used to do quite often – for example, if you used to have a date night each week – and you're not doing that any more, really try to rebuild that connection with them, doing things that you enjoy together.

That includes having sex. If you enjoyed having sex with your partner before you were trying to conceive, and suddenly it's turned into a massive obligation in your month, try having sex for fun again. Change the way you perceive it. Try having sex just to connect and feel emotionally close to your partner.

If it's all getting too much, think about taking a little break from trying to conceive – see it as a kind of conception holiday.

There will, of course, be circumstances in which there's a medical reason behind the fact that you're not pregnant, and you will need to seek professional help. I have friends that this has happened to, and sometimes it's been hard to know how to support them or what the best thing to say or do is. But what helped me was to just ask them: 'How can I support you? What do you need me to do or say?'

The online fertility community IVF Babble was set up by two women, Sara Marshall-Page and Tracey Bambrough, who have each had long, complicated and emotional fertility journeys. They wanted to do something to help others facing the same daunting experience and decided to create a resource that did not yet exist: a resource packed full of trusted information from top fertility experts, where men and women across the world could come and learn more about their fertility and their options, and which would help them navigate their way through their treatment.

They also wanted to break down the stigma of shame attached to infertility by starting conversations and sharing real stories of other people going through the same thing. When it came

to writing a guide to what to do if you are navigating this situation, I knew there was nobody better placed to reassure you that you are not alone and to offer you an overview of what to do next.

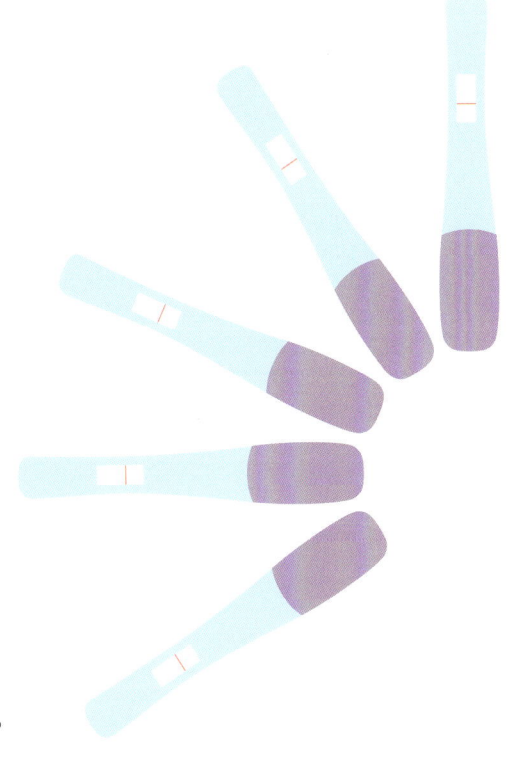

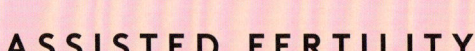

ASSISTED FERTILITY

IVF Babble

If you're trying to conceive (TTC) and things are taking longer than you'd expected or hoped, it can become one of the most stressful and upsetting times in your life. It can be all-consuming as you enter a world of advice – both solicited or, as is too often the case, unsolicited (well meaning or otherwise). Old wives' tales and unsubstantiated 'tricks' to become pregnant abound, and often this can leave us feeling lonely, isolated and like there's something we're not doing right (trust us, you're doing everything you should be).

TTC – WHEN SHOULD I SPEAK TO MY DOCTOR?

Knowing when to start asking for help is an important step in getting access to assisted fertility treatments and discovering what options may be available to you.

It's generally accepted that if you haven't become pregnant after a year of trying (this means having unprotected sex regularly, every two to three days) and you're female and under 35 years old, you should speak to your GP. If you have a health condition that means you may struggle to become pregnant, or you're 35 years old or over, you should make an appointment sooner.

Your GP will ask you questions about your and your partner's medical histories and how long you've been trying to become pregnant. They will also take your age into account. As a woman ages, her chances of becoming pregnant begin to fall, particularly once she's reached her mid to late 30s. Male fertility can also decline with age.

Given all this information, they can then provide advice on your options and your potential chances of having a family, and will then refer you to a specialist for further tests, investigations and treatments. Conception is a shared responsibility, so it's essential for both partners to consult with a specialist.

IVF, or in vitro fertilisation – one of the more common types of assisted fertility – is only offered on the NHS in certain areas of the UK, and will depend on strict criteria, including your age and health. Your GP will be able to inform you of the funding available in your area.

People in the LGBTQ+ community should speak to a specialist once they've decided that they wish to start their journey to parenthood.

POSSIBLE REASONS FOR INFERTILITY

In women, infertility can be caused by a number of health conditions that affect the reproductive organs. These include polycystic ovary syndrome (PCOS), endometriosis, fibroids, pelvic inflammatory disease and premature ovarian failure. These conditions all have different symptoms, causes and treatments, but if you have difficult, painful periods, heavy bleeding, irregular periods, pelvic pain or anything else that bothers you regarding your reproductive health, it's important to speak to a doctor in order to get a diagnosis to increase your chances of treatment and a successful pregnancy.

Some medications, such as those used to treat cancer, inflammation and psychosis, can also affect fertility. Alcohol abuse and illegal drug use can also make it more difficult to become pregnant.

Male infertility is often caused by a low sperm count and quality, and can also be caused by certain medications, including chemotherapy and radiotherapy drugs, those to manage inflammation and anabolic steroids. Illegal drugs and alcohol can also reduce sperm quality. Testicular problems, such as injury, infections and defects that you may have been born with can also interfere with your ability to become a parent.

Age is also a significant factor, especially in women, as the number and quality of your eggs reduces over time. This is something that can also affect sperm health.

Unexplained infertility, with no obvious cause, also accounts for around a quarter of all cases. However, starting the conversation with your GP can mean that assisted fertility techniques can help you.

WHAT TYPES OF ASSISTED FERTILITY TREATMENTS ARE AVAILABLE?

The type of assisted fertility available to you will depend on your age, gender, medical history, reproductive health and whether you're embarking on this journey on your own or with a partner. If it is with a partner, the type of assistance will also depend on their medical history and reproductive health. Your specialist will first perform tests to ascertain your reproductive health, including tests on your/your partner's eggs and womb and/or sperm if necessary.

— IVF is an option for both straight and same-sex couples and for those wanting to enter parenthood alone. Depending on your gender and reproductive health, IVF can be performed using your eggs and sperm or donated eggs and/or sperm.

— Intrauterine insemination (IUI), also known as artificial insemination, is a fertility treatment that involves selecting and injecting high-quality sperm directly into a woman's uterus. This method can use either a partner's sperm or donor sperm and is suitable for individuals needing donated sperm, couples facing difficulties with vaginal intercourse, or those requiring specific assistance to achieve a safe pregnancy. While IUI is less invasive and more affordable than IVF, it typically has lower success rates, as it relies on the body's natural processes for fertilisation. IUI may not be appropriate for individuals with significant fertility issues, such as blocked fallopian tubes or severe endometriosis, especially as age increases.

— Surrogacy is also an option for those who cannot carry a pregnancy for medical reasons or for gay men wishing to become parents. Again, surrogacy can involve your own eggs and/or sperm, or donated eggs and/or sperm.

THE FINANCIAL IMPLICATIONS OF ASSISTED FERTILITY

Sadly, the days of NHS-funded IVF are fast disappearing, but that doesn't mean it has to be out of your grasp if you don't have the money to fund it yourself. Private clinics will usually offer some kind of finance deal. IVF refund programmes are a supportive treatment option that provide a set price for several IVF cycles, or even unlimited ones. If a baby doesn't arrive, you may receive a refund, with the amount and specific terms varying based on the programme. Factors such as your age and the number of cycles included can influence these details. Other financial options are personal loans, insurance and grants. However, it's very important to keep in mind that IVF and other assisted fertility techniques are expensive. Costs vary around the country, but one cycle of IVF costs on average around £5,000 and can be as much as £13,000. Having more than one cycle and/or paying for the storage of frozen embryos means that the total cost can run into tens of thousands of pounds.

THE POSSIBLE EMOTIONAL, PHYSICAL AND MENTAL HEALTH CHALLENGES

Infertility and fertility treatments take a toll not only on our finances, but also on our physical and mental health. The most obvious challenge to any assisted fertility process is how you'll feel if things don't work out. Being told to stay positive is perhaps one of the most frustrating things about a less-than-straightforward route to parenthood. We get it. When you're in the midst of hormonal surges, medical bills and all of the 'what ifs', keeping a positive mindset is hard. But with the right support, you can make your way through this journey feeling as positive as possible, to help manage the emotional toll.

Procedures such as IVF involve injections and other practices that can also be physically gruelling. Support from your loved ones, employer and medical team are all essential. Platforms like IVF Babble can help you find this support.

WAYS TO PRESERVE YOUR FERTILITY

Perhaps right now, having a family isn't part of your immediate plans, or you may be concerned about your future fertility. Either way, there are fertility preservation procedures that can help you put your fertility on pause. These include egg and sperm freezing, and freezing embryos created with your partner or with donated eggs and/or sperm.

HOW IVF BABBLE CAN HELP

IVF Babble is run by people who have been on assisted fertility journeys. They understand every emotion, question and fear running through your mind. They can help you navigate all of it, from which route to take to parenthood, to how to manage the financial side, and what the future can look like if things don't end the way you'd hoped.

Visit IVFbabble.com for more information.

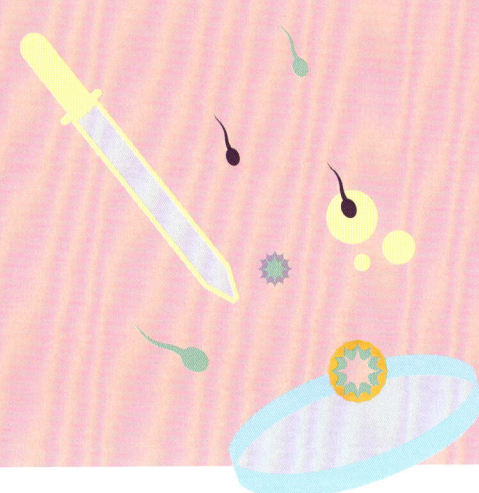

FREEZING YOUR EGGS

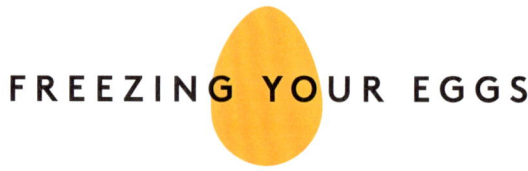

Egg freezing, or oocyte cryopreservation, is a process that allows women to preserve their eggs for use in the future. It involves collecting your eggs, freezing them, and then thawing them later when you're ready to pursue pregnancy. It's a way to take control of your fertility and timeframe for getting pregnant, especially since a woman's chances of conceiving naturally decline as we age due to the decrease in both the quality and quantity of our eggs.

WHO SHOULD CONSIDER EGG FREEZING?

You might be wondering whether it's the right path for you, so here are some scenarios where egg freezing could be a viable option:

Medical Reasons: If you're facing medical treatments, such as chemotherapy or radiotherapy, which could impact your fertility, egg freezing allows you to safeguard your eggs before treatment begins.

Personal Choice: You're not quite ready to start a family but concerned about age-related fertility decline? Choosing to freeze your eggs allow you to pause your biological clock, giving you more time to make the decision that's right for you.

Occupational Risks: Certain professions come with higher risks so egg freezing can be a precautionary measure to preserve fertility.

Gender Transitioning: For those transitioning from female to male, preserving fertility before starting hormone therapy or undergoing surgery is an important consideration.

THE EGG FREEZING PROCESS

Egg freezing will involve several key steps:

1 **Initial Assessment:** You'll undergo tests for infectious diseases like HIV and hepatitis. This doesn't affect your eligibility but ensures that all samples are stored safely.

2 **Ovarian Stimulation:** Over two to three weeks, you'll take hormonal medications to stimulate your ovaries to produce multiple eggs.

3 **Egg Retrieval:** Once your eggs are ready, they're collected under sedation or general anaesthetic.

4 **Freezing:** A cryoprotectant is added to protect the eggs during the freezing process, which is typically done through vitrification, a rapid freezing method that has been shown to have higher success rates.

5 **Storage:** Your frozen eggs are stored in liquid nitrogen tanks until you're ready to use them.

6 **Thawing and Fertilisation:** When the time comes, the eggs are thawed and fertilised with sperm, either from

a partner or a donor, before being transferred to your uterus.

SUCCESS RATES AND CONSIDERATIONS

While it sounds like a brilliant solution, it's really important to approach egg freezing with realistic expectations. Success rates can vary, based on factors such as age at the time of freezing and the number of eggs retrieved. Younger women generally have higher success rates, as egg quality tends to decline with age.

COSTS AND FUNDING

The financial aspect is a big consideration. There is the initial cost of the procedure and then the annual storage, so you need to get really good advice and make sure you check out all of your options. In the UK, NHS funding may be available, particularly if you're undergoing medical treatments that could affect your fertility, but this varies depending on where you live.

CONSIDERATIONS

As with any medical procedure, egg freezing carries potential risks, including:

Ovarian Hyperstimulation Syndrome (OHSS): A condition where the ovaries over-respond to stimulation, leading to swelling and pain.

Complications from egg retrieval: Though rare, there can be risks associated with the surgical procedure used to collect eggs.

Please, please have a chat to your healthcare provider to understand the risks and help you navigate the challenges. Deciding to freeze your eggs is a hugely personal choice, impacted by your life goals, health and circumstances. It's not an insurance policy for future pregnancy, but it does offer you an opportunity to extend your fertility window. If you're considering egg freezing, please do consult a fertility specialist to discuss your options, understand the process, and make the decision that's right for you.

YOUR STORIES

'Single by chance, I've been doing IVF solo, in a conscious way I feel really proud of.' — Sarah

So far I've lost 7 embryos. As single women aren't supported by the NHS, I currently can't afford more rounds. But I'm hopeful that one day I'll get to be the mum I feel I am. In the meantime, I'm living that energy.

Davina: Sarah, I'm so happy for you doing IVF in a conscious way. I love that expression and the way that it's made you feel. I'm so pleased you're on this journey and really, really good luck.

YOUR STORIES

'I'm a British-born Sikh with a traditional mother. I met my Caucasian husband when we were both 42. I tried to get pregnant naturally but knew we had to check things out.' — Satvere

There were no issues except age. The donor route was suggested but I knew it wouldn't be easy to find an Indian donor as it is not the done thing in the community. We tried five rounds of IVF with my own eggs but had no success. We still wanted a family and I wanted to be pregnant so I had to grieve the loss of my genetics and get my head around donor conception. Time was not on our side at 46, so we went for a Caucasian donor, something my family had to come on board with.

We had our boy on the first attempt, at 46. We tried to give him a sibling. On the fifth attempt, having been diagnosed perimenopausal, I gave birth to a boy and girl twin at 48. Great pregnancies. The kids are now almost 7 and 5 and I'm trying to keep fit and healthy for them. They are our babies and even though they don't look like me, they have many of my traits. I occasionally grieve my loss but these beauties are what my kids were meant to be.

Davina: Wow, Satvere, you and your partner have gone on quite a journey. Thanks so much for sharing this with us. It's incredibly hard losing so many pregnancies, but you got your wonderful family. Congratulations and lots of love.

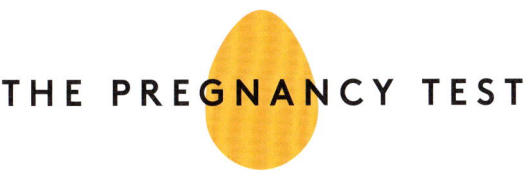

THE PREGNANCY TEST

If you've been trying for a baby for a while, you're likely going to be hyper aware of any changes in your body or how you're feeling and will be looking out for the tiniest indication you're pregnant. I remember that my sense of smell suddenly became really acute – windscreen washer was a particularly offensive one, weirdly, but there are lots of general signs that it's time to take that pregnancy test if you haven't already. These are the most common:

— Your period is late or you've missed it (this is obviously easier to track if you've got a fairly regular cycle).

— You're feeling sick or abnormally tired (morning sickness usually kicks in when you're about four to six weeks pregnant).

— You're weeing more often.

— You suddenly develop constipation.

— Your boobs are swollen or feel sore or tender.

— Some foods start to taste weird, or you've developed strong cravings.

You can buy pregnancy tests from pharmacists and some supermarkets. You might also be able to get a test free from your GP. The tests can give a quick result and you can do the test in private. Taking the test can be laden with pressure and anticipation and may feel really nerve-wracking. Some people do tests on their own, others choose to do it with their partners or friends present. Think long and hard before filming it for social media.

It can be a big moment so before you do it, have a think about any support you might want around you if you feel you'll need it.

If you do a test and it's positive, then as long as you've followed the packet instructions to the letter, it's likely you are definitely pregnant. Negative tests can be a bit of a grey area. I really don't want to give anybody false hope by saying this, but when I was trying for a baby, I did a pregnancy test and it came up negative. I had some spotting two days later and got quite sad about it, but two days after that the spotting stopped, I did another test and I was pregnant. I'm telling you this because science shows that sometimes your hormones behave quite strangely around the time of conception. Midwives I've spoken to confirm that my experience can be quite common, so if you do have a negative test, it might be worth waiting a week if you still haven't had a proper period and testing again to make sure.

If you think you might be pregnant but still get a negative result and your period hasn't arrived, speak to your GP.

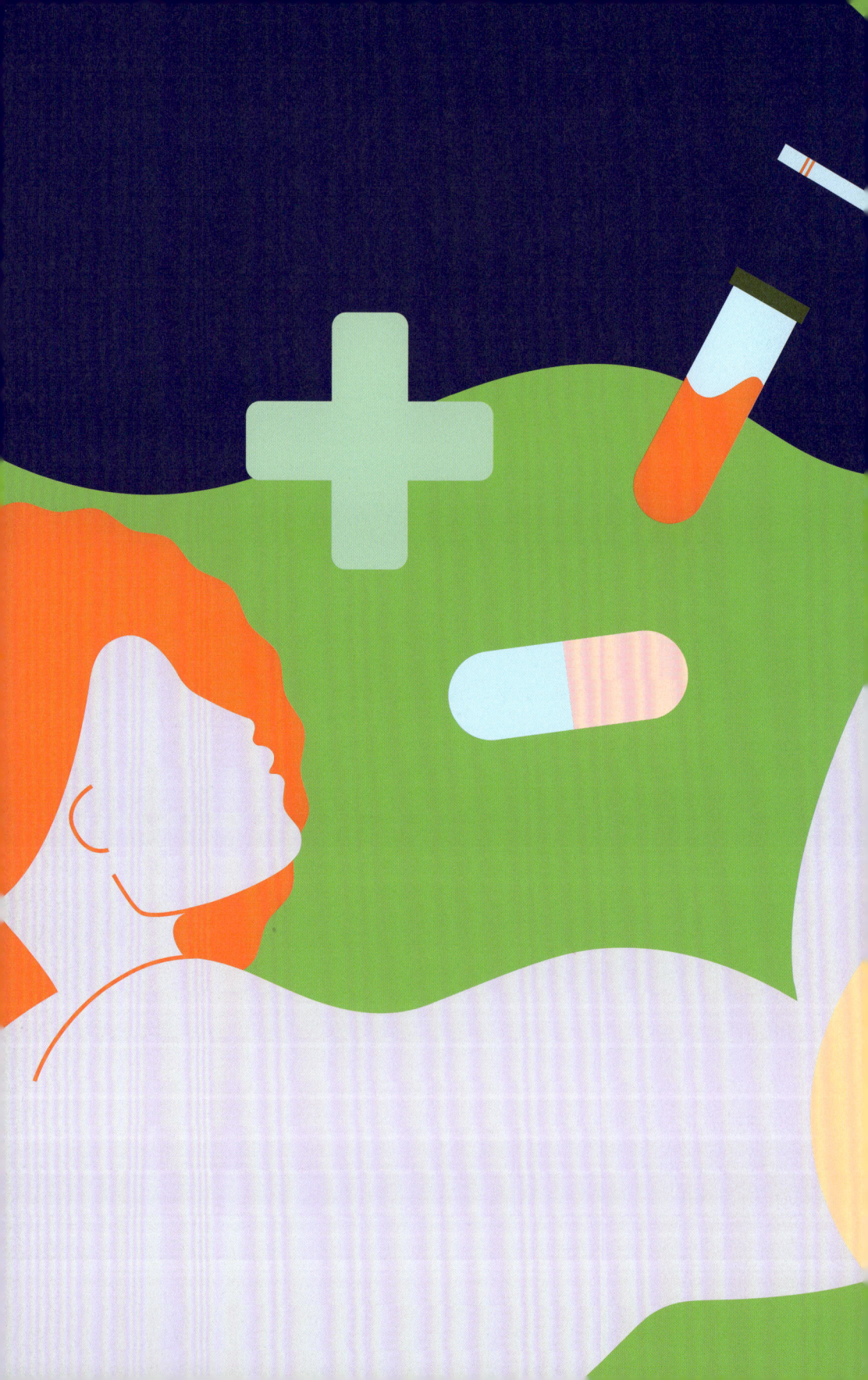

CHAPTER 2

FIRST TRIMESTER

0–12 WEEKS

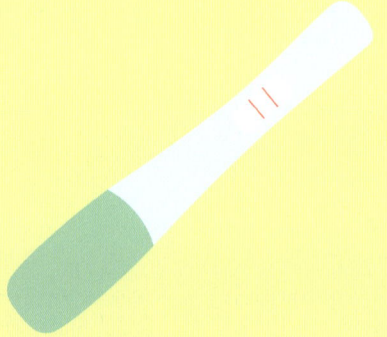

Your test is positive!

YOU'VE GOT THE LITTLE COLOURED LINE – WHAT NEXT?

Seeing that coloured line appear on your pregnancy test is one of the most exciting, terrifying, overwhelming and indescribable feelings in the world. It's life-changing. You might want to scream about it and tell everyone straight away, and a million different questions and thoughts will probably be flying around your head. And some of you might be confused about what to do next. I wanted to know when my due date was. I was thinking about telling my husband, my family, my work, but I was also just trying to imagine what the next nine months were going to look and feel like.

The first thing you need to do is book yourself in for antenatal care. Previously, you had to book yourself in via your GP, but nowadays you can just look up your local NHS Trust and self-refer by filling in a form on the hospital's website. If you have any questions or doubts, just call the maternity hospital and speak to them.

Life, and how you look after yourself, changes from this point onwards, so for this chapter we've asked Dr Federica Amati from the ZOE team to talk about your nutritional needs during this trimester (see page 66). One of the other things you'll need to think about is supplements, as it's recommended that you take 400 micrograms of folic acid every day from when you start trying for a baby until you're 12 weeks pregnant.[15] It's difficult to get the amount of folic acid recommended for a healthy pregnancy just from food, which is why it's important to take a supplement. Folic acid can help prevent birth defects, including spina bifida, so if you weren't taking it before, you should start as soon as you find out you're pregnant.

You might also be eligible for free pregnancy and breastfeeding vitamin supplements, as well as help to buy milk, fruit and vegetables and other foods for you and your child until your child turns four as part of the NHS Healthy Start scheme, so do visit healthystart.nhs.uk to find out all the details.

Seeing that coloured line appear on your pregnancy test is one of the most exciting, terrifying, overwhelming and indescribable feelings in the world.

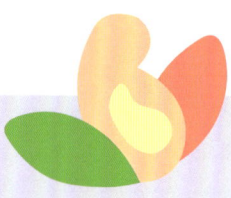

ANTENATAL CARE

Midwife Marley

Finding out you're pregnant will prompt such a mixture of emotions. Believe me, I know – like Davina, I have been there several times! You should inform your care provider as soon as you get a positive pregnancy test, so that you can be booked in for antenatal care, discuss your birthplace options with a midwife and get access to important screening tests. Regardless of whether you are considering a home birth, a birth-centre birth or a hospital birth, booking in to your local hospital to receive care is usually the first step. Some people decide to opt for independent or private midwifery care but will still attend the hospital during pregnancy for ultrasound scans or blood tests.

When the hospital receives your referral, you will be sent a booking appointment with the midwife. Depending on the information given on the referral form, this may be held at your local GP surgery, or within the antenatal clinic at the hospital. The booking appointment should be held somewhere between the eighth and twelfth week of pregnancy, so it's important that you complete the self-referral as soon as possible. This appointment is usually the longest and includes your medical and social history, past pregnancy history (if applicable), blood tests, urine test and a blood-pressure check. The blood test offered is to check for your blood group and antibodies, HIV, syphilis, hepatitis B, sickle cell, thalassaemia and glucose levels. Although they are recommended, you can opt out of any of these tests.

This appointment is a good time to ask any burning questions you may have about your care. If, after going through your history, the midwife determines you would benefit from seeing an obstetric doctor (for example, if you have a history of heart problems or diabetes), a referral will be made, with your consent.

WHO'S GOING
TO BE LOOKING AFTER YOU?

Depending on whether you are being looked after by the NHS or privately, you're going to be seeing a variety of people over the course of your pregnancy: your GP, a health visitor, a sonographer, a midwife or midwives, and possibly an obstetrician if your pregnancy has been classed as 'complicated'. There may be others, too, depending on your individual needs – an anaesthetist, an obstetric physiotherapist or a nutritionist, for example.

Your GP will look after anything that's not related to your baby as they would normally. Your health visitor will be a trained nurse and they are the person you'll see after your baby is born, as they do the postnatal check-ups, but they might also come and introduce themselves before the birth. A sonographer will carry out your scans. Your midwife (or midwives) is the person you're going to be seeing the most, right through your pregnancy, labour and birth, and even after the birth. Overleaf Marley has explained exactly what it is they do.

I was incredibly lucky to be able to go down the private midwife route – it meant that I had an independent midwife, so I saw Caroline throughout my entire first pregnancy, and then Pam, too, when the time came to deliver Holly. If you're being looked after by the NHS, your hospital will do its best to ensure continuity of care; ideally you'll have the same midwife and care team looking after you throughout your pregnancy so that they can get to know you and your birth plan. But as we know, the health service is stretched and incredibly busy, so that's not always possible. If you're worried about seeing lots of different people through your pregnancy, don't be afraid to speak up. You can ask your midwife about it at your first appointment and check whether you're likely to be seeing just them, or others as well. Seeing the same person is going to be more likely if you're giving birth in a midwife-led centre or at home.

Midwives truly are the most amazing people. Their experience and deep understanding of birth means that they can instinctively tell what's going on in your body. I was always amazed at how they can anticipate signs of your labour's progression just by noticing a shift in your breathing pattern or the noises you're making – but they're also there to support you and advocate for you. I still feel so lucky to have met Caroline and Pam. Knowing them both well made me feel safe and reassured that everything would be okay. Pam sadly died a couple of years ago, but she remains such an important figure to me and my kids because of the impact she had on our lives by being present at each of their births.

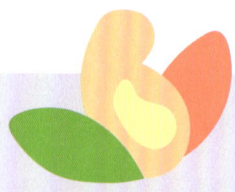

WHAT IS A MIDWIFE?

Midwife Marley

In the UK, a midwife plays a crucial role in providing care and support to women throughout pregnancy, childbirth and the postnatal period. The term 'midwife' originates from Old English, meaning 'with woman', highlighting the integral partnership between the midwife and the mother-to-be.

Although the vast majority of midwives are female, there are many male midwives too, which shows that midwifery is not a gendered role.

During pregnancy, a midwife offers comprehensive antenatal care, which includes regular check-ups to monitor the health of both mother and baby. They carry out physical examinations, such as measuring blood pressure and checking the baby's growth, as well as providing advice on nutrition, exercise and preparation for childbirth. Midwives also offer emotional support, addressing any concerns or anxieties the mother may have, and empowering her to make informed decisions about her pregnancy and birth plan (we

explain all about what this is on page 91). Midwives work closely with a wider, multi-disciplinary team, including obstetric doctors, physiotherapists, neonatal nurses, children's services, GPs and health visitors.

When labour begins, midwives play a supportive role in the birth process. They offer the mother reassurance, comfort measures and guidance on breathing and relaxation techniques. At the same time, they monitor the progress of labour, assessing the mother's and baby's wellbeing and facilitating appropriate medical interventions if necessary. They should advocate for the woman's preferences and ensure that her wishes are respected throughout the birthing experience, whether she chooses to give birth at a hospital, a birthing centre or at home.

Midwives are trained to assist women in various birthing scenarios, including straightforward physiological births, water births, home births and births with medical interventions, such as epidurals or caesarean sections but they are not surgeons, so they don't carry out caesareans themselves. They can perform a supportive role in theatre if surgery is required, such as by placing a catheter in the bladder, keeping the mother calm and sometimes passing the surgeon tools to perform the caesarean. They are also handed the baby once it is born, and will check it over, sometimes along with a neonatal doctor if it's an emergency.

Midwives have the skills and knowledge to manage complications that may arise during labour, working collaboratively with obstetricians and other healthcare professionals to ensure the safety and wellbeing of mother and baby. They can identify when complications arise. In these situations, an obstetric doctor may be called in to provide care with support from the midwife. Following birth, midwives continue to provide care and support during the postnatal period at home and in the community. They offer guidance on breastfeeding, newborn care and maternal recovery, conducting regular postnatal visits to monitor the health and progress of both mother and baby. Midwives also provide emotional support, addressing any concerns or challenges the mother may encounter as she adjusts to parenthood.

Midwives are dedicated healthcare professionals who should prioritise the physical, emotional and psychological wellbeing of women throughout the journey of pregnancy, childbirth and the postnatal period. Their holistic approach emphasises personalised care and support, to empower women to make informed choices about their maternity care.

YOUR STORIES

'My midwife was ace. I thank my lucky stars for having her with me for nine months.' — Elle

'I was frightened of birth. I think many of us are subconsciously taught to fear it.' — Elle

I was extremely lucky that I opted for a continuity-of-care package with my midwife, Sheriden – 'Beyoncé' to me. As our relationship progressed and her caring, nurturing ways started to reframe my ideas of pregnancy and birth, I found myself challenging myself to look into all my options and researching how our bodies and babies work. What environment are we meant to birth in? What positions can we birth in? What hormones support or surprise birth? What do we need when we've given birth to support us in our recovery? To my surprise, I did a complete 180. I went from wanting a very medicalised/ planned hospital birth to opting for a home birth. My midwife was ace: 'Well,

if you don't fancy it on the day, you just go and give birth where you want. This is your body and baby, you do what you feel is best. You've got this,' she'd say. I thank my lucky stars for having her with me for nine months.

Davina: Well, Beyoncé sounds like an absolute legend, Elle – I'm so glad you found somebody like her. Midwives are amazing. And as somebody who did the same thing as you and totally changed my mind about the type of birth I wanted, I can absolutely relate to how meeting somebody you trust and feeling supported by them can help alter your birthing experience. We all need a Beyoncé at our births.

'I had hyperemesis gravidarum with both my pregnancies.' — Christie

I was so unwell in my first pregnancy that it took me six years to decide to have a second child. My second pregnancy was even worse and had it not been for Covid I would have been hospitalised. Completely bedridden, unable to eat or drink even water for months. I feel this is an underrepresented part of pregnancy as I don't think people understood the full

severity of it. There is a great Instagram account called @HGSUPPORTUK that has loads of info.

Davina: Thank you, Christie, for sharing your experience of HG and for the account. I know so many people are put off from having another baby because of it. This is really helpful.

IS YOUR PREGNANCY CONSIDERED 'STRAIGHTFORWARD' OR 'COMPLEX'?

At some point during your pregnancy, most likely at your first appointment with your midwife when they go through your medical history, your pregnancy may be classed as 'complex' or 'high risk', as opposed to a straightforward or low-risk pregnancy. Although I know it sounds a bit scary, it just means that you'll be offered closer monitoring from an obstetrician who has expertise in addressing potential complications and can intervene with treatments and procedures when necessary. Below are some of the main reasons why your pregnancy might be considered complex:

— Pregnant with twins
  or multiple babies

— Aged over 40 or under 18

— Significantly overweight
  or underweight

— Previous caesarean

— Previous postpartum haemorrhage
  (heavy bleeding after birth,
  requiring treatment such as
  a blood transfusion)

— Previous shoulder dystocia
  (difficulty in delivery the shoulders)

— Previous preterm birth
  (before 37 weeks)

— Previous pre-eclampsia
  or eclampsia

— Previous retained placenta

— Previous stillbirth

— Pre-existing diabetes

— Pre-existing heart disease

— History of high blood
  pressure or stroke

— Pre-existing epilepsy

— Some mental health conditions
  requiring inpatient care[16]

Each of these has its own implications for your pregnancy, such as additional scans, seeing a specialist or being advised to have a caesarean, so it's just good to be aware of your status so that you can assess the risks and use that knowledge to help inform your decisions – it may, though not always, affect your birth plan.

SCANS AND SCREENING

Every time I went for a scan or test, I would get quite nervous. I was hoping the doctor would be able to find the baby's heartbeat; that the scans would be fine. I was worried about whether my baby was okay; whether there was a complication. I would always be thinking, *What do I do if there is a problem?* As I've said, I was generally quite anxious during my first pregnancy – you might be much calmer, but I would still really recommend that when you go to any kind of appointment, you take someone with you, as this can help calm any anxiety or nerves. My pregnancies were smooth and there weren't any red flags at any point, but I've had friends who have been told something difficult alone – and I know it would have been much easier for them to cope with if somebody had been there to support them through that. It doesn't necessarily have to be a partner; it could be your mum or a friend, but do try to go with someone.

Marley has outlined opposite what appointments you will be invited to attend throughout your pregnancy, which includes two scans – your dating scan at around 12 weeks, and your screening scan at around 20 weeks. You don't have to have these scans, and your choice will be respected if that's what you decide; you'll still get looked after by the NHS. You'll also be able to have a chat with your medical team before you make your decision.

> I would still really recommend that when you go to any kind of appointment, you take someone with you, as this can help calm any anxiety or nerves.

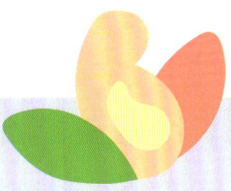

YOUR ANTENATAL APPOINTMENTS

Midwife Marley

During the first trimester, it's a good idea to plan ahead and get an understanding of when you should be seeing your midwife throughout your pregnancy. I've put together a schedule that you can refer to at any time:

11–14 WEEKS

Ultrasound scan at the maternity unit to confirm your approximate gestation – your due date, and screening test for chromosomal anomalies such as Patau syndrome, Edwards syndrome and Down syndrome. Patau syndrome is a rare genetic disorder in which babies can have a wide range of health problems. Their growth in the womb is often restricted, resulting in a low birth weight, and 8 out of 10 will be born with severe heart defects. In many cases, development is so restricted that it results in miscarriage, stillbirth or the baby dying shortly after birth. Edwards syndrome is another genetic condition, caused by an extra chromosome in the body's cells that causes low birth

weight, ears in a low position on the baby's head, cleft lip or palate, club foot, problems with their heart, kidneys or spine and breathing or digestion. Down syndrome is a genetic condition caused when an unusual cell division results in an extra full or partial copy of a chromosome. Screening is carried out by chorionic villus sampling (CVS) – cells taken from the placenta –or amniocentesis whereby a needle is passed into the abdomen to collect amniotic fluid. This enables the lab to extract the baby's DNA and test for any of the above conditions conclusively.

This detailed ultrasound measures the thickness of the skin at the back of your baby's neck, known as the nuchal translucency (NT) measurement. This measurement, along with other factors such as your age, the baby's gestational age, and certain biochemical markers in your blood (specifically, the levels of two proteins and a hormone), are all taken into consideration when assessing the risk for these chromosomal abnormalities. If the chance of having a baby with one of the conditions above is high, you should be notified within a few days. If it is low, a letter usually arrives to inform you within a couple of weeks.

It's important to know that this test doesn't provide a definitive diagnosis but rather helps to identify those who may benefit from further testing, such as the NIPT test (another more accurate blood test), chorionic villus sampling (CVS) or amniocentesis.

16 WEEKS

Your first antenatal appointment with the midwife to check on your wellbeing and to discuss your initial antenatal screening results. During this appointment you will also have your urine tested to check for infections and high sugar, which can be a sign of gestational diabetes, and you'll have your blood pressure taken.

19–21 WEEKS

You'll have an anomaly ultrasound scan to check that all major structures of the baby are developing normally. This scan is a pretty detailed one and the appointment lasts for around 30 minutes. Some people like to find out the sex of the baby at this point although it's not always possible.

25 WEEKS (FIRST-TIME MUMS)

It will have been a while since you would have seen a midwife so this routine appointment is another good time to ask questions you may have about your pregnancy. During this brief appointment, the midwife will check your urine and blood pressure, and measure your bump. They will also ask you about your baby's movements, which probably won't have formed a regular pattern just yet.

28 WEEKS

Routine antenatal appointment with the midwife. They will check everything they checked at the previous appointment and will also offer a blood test to check your iron levels, glucose levels, and to see if any antibodies have developed in your blood. If it was determined at your booking appointment that you were at high risk for gestational diabetes, a separate test called the glucose tolerance test (GTT) will be offered at this stage too.

31 WEEKS (FIRST-TIME MUMS)

If you're a first-time mum you'll have a routine antenatal appointment as a 'check-in'. The midwife will check your urine, blood pressure and bump measurement, along with feeling your

abdomen with their hands to see whether your baby is lying head down, bottom down, or across your belly.

34 WEEKS

This appointment is a good time to discuss your birth preferences or birth plan (see page 91). The midwife will carry out the same examinations as the 31-week appointment and if they feel the baby isn't head down yet, you'll be offered an ultrasound to check. If your iron levels were low at your 28-week appointment, they may recheck them at this stage.

36, 38 AND 40 WEEKS

These appointments are routine check-ins for your blood pressure, urine, bump measurement and to identify your baby's position. At 40 weeks if you haven't gone into labour, there may be some discussion about you being induced (see page 197).

41 WEEKS

At this point you're probably wondering when the baby will arrive! You'll also probably be feeling heavy and tired. You've not got much longer to go though. During this appointment the midwife will carry out the same checks as the previous one. They will ensure you have the contact details for the midwives if you've opted for a home birth and the maternity team if you're planning on giving birth in a birth centre or hospital.

42+ WEEKS

Although many women will opt to be induced at this point, some do not. If your baby has not yet come to say hello, your maternity team will still want to keep an eye on the wellbeing of you and your baby. You will continue to be offered antenatal appointments at more regular intervals until your baby makes an appearance.

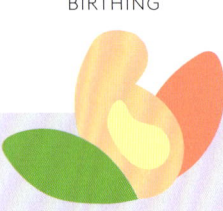

TWINS AND MULTIPLES

Midwife Marley

Perhaps you've discovered at your first scan that you're having more than one baby. Well, if so, you'll be joining the 1.5 per cent of expectant parents in the UK who are welcoming twins, triplets or more. It can certainly be a shock to discover you're having more than one baby – I remember the feeling well when I had my twins. Many questions may run through your mind: *How will it affect me physically? What will the birth be like? How will we afford it?* If you have these thoughts, you're not alone; having two or more babies at once is a big deal! But there are plenty of organisations that can support you, such as Twins Trust (formerly TAMBA).

There are many differences during pregnancy and birth when having multiples; for example, you are more likely to experience more severe morning sickness than if you were expecting one baby. This is due to the higher level of pregnancy hormones secreted by the placenta. Weight gain will usually be more rapid, and your bump will grow more quickly. You'll probably feel more tired, and your appetite is likely to be through the

roof! As there is more than one baby wriggling around, foetal movements may seem constant, but you will likely soon work out which baby is moving at a given time.

Although most multiple births are unproblematic, they do come with a higher chance of complications, such as maternal gestational diabetes, pre-eclampsia, preterm birth and placenta issues. For this reason, antenatal appointments for multiples tend to be more frequent, as are ultrasound scans. Identical babies who share an amniotic sac and placenta are at greater risk of developing complications, such as twin-to-twin transfusion syndrome (TTTS). This is when there is an imbalance in blood flow from the placenta to the twins, resulting in one twin getting more than the other. Babies with TTTS are carefully monitored and early birth is usually anticipated.

Preterm birth is common with multiples: around 60 per cent of twins are born before 37 weeks, and around 80 per cent of triplets are born before 35 weeks. Early birth via induction of

labour or caesarean section will be discussed depending on the number, type and wellbeing of the multiple babies, and taking into consideration your own preferences.

It is often assumed that having more than one baby means that a caesarean is always warranted. This isn't true. Many people carrying twins who have experienced an uncomplicated pregnancy will go on to give birth vaginally with no issues. It's also a misconception that it is more painful with two; the contractions will feel no different to having one baby on board. The only difference is that once one baby is born, the pushing stage begins again for the next. Many second twins will follow soon after the birth of their sibling. If you are planning on having a vaginal birth, the position of the first twin (the one sitting lowest in the uterus) will be considered. A vaginal birth is more favourable if the first twin is head down and there are no other factors that would indicate a caesarean being recommended. It is worth bearing in mind that there is a chance that an assisted birth with forceps or ventouse (vacuum cup) may be suggested for the second twin if there is an obstruction, and, at times, a caesarean for the second twin if they are not able to be born vaginally. These factors will be discussed in depth with your obstetric doctor. Triplets and high

multiples are less likely to be born vaginally, although it's not unheard of.

As many multiples are born early, they may spend time in the neonatal intensive care unit (NICU) while they grow stronger, as many are born with a low birth weight and may need assistance with breathing. You may get the chance to visit the NICU or speak to someone from the neonatal team prior to the birth if you would like to but this isn't a must. It's worth noting that not all multiples are born early. There have been cases where twins have reached full term before labour begins and have left the hospital with no neonatal stay.

FEELING SICK
(AKA THE PUKE-A-THON BEGINS)

The first thing to know about the famous 'morning sickness' we've all heard pregnant women talk about is that, despite its name, the feelings of nausea and vomiting can strike at any time of day (they're just more common in the morning). And the second thing is that it can start early on in your pregnancy. My morning sickness began pretty much a few days after I found out I was pregnant and went on until around 14 weeks. For most women it generally settles by 16 to 20 weeks, and basically it's all to do with your pregnancy hormones going mad, so there's no way of knowing whether or how it will affect you. Some women don't suffer from it at all; some just feel nauseous; some will have vomiting, too.

I was really anxious about the effect that being sick would have on my baby, but apparently there's no evidence that it affects them at all.

Everyone will have different ways of coping with the feeling of sickness – sometimes it's simply a case of sticking it out, but the main thing that helped me was eating. Instead of having three big meals each day, I found that eating little meals more often eased my symptoms. Resting and just taking it a bit easier (I was SO tired during the first trimester) also meant that I felt less sick. But other people will tell you that acupuncture, anti-nausea tablets or the wristbands you wear for travel sickness can help. Having really bland, plain snacks, like crackers or dry toast, nearby was also helpful for me because my sense of smell became so powerful – strong smells made me feel sick, too. But it's really a case of trying things to see what works for you. Some women keep dry snacks by their bed as they start to feel sick as soon as they wake up, and that helps ease the sickness a little.

Severe morning sickness is called hyperemesis gravidarum (HG), and Marley is going to explain what that is. It can be very, very serious because it becomes so hard to keep any fluid in your body. If you suffer from HG, you might need to speak to your midwife or your doctor about getting some specialist treatment. There are also charities that can give you a bit of advice and support with morning sickness, including Pregnancy Sickness Support, so if you're worried about it or want some help navigating it, do reach out to them.

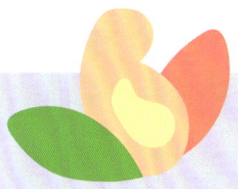

HYPEREMESIS GRAVIDARUM

Midwife Marley

While nausea and sporadic vomiting are typical symptoms of morning sickness in the early stages of pregnancy, more severe symptoms, such as frequent vomiting, are classified as hyperemesis gravidarum (HG), a crippling illness that can occur throughout pregnancy. HG is diagnosed when someone vomits at least five times a day. The vast majority of sufferers report being unable to keep anything down, vomiting 30 to 40 times or more daily, even when their stomachs are empty. HG affects around 1 per cent of women in the UK and can take its toll physically and mentally. Weight loss can occur, along with the depletion of vitamin K and electrolyte imbalances, so hospital care is frequently necessary to control symptoms and avoid dehydration.

Many sufferers will spend long bouts of their pregnancy in and out of the hospital, being prescribed medications to help combat the sickness.

Sometimes these medicines work, but sadly sometimes they aren't effective. It's not unusual for someone with severe HG to also be administered a drip to replenish fluid loss from excessive vomiting.

It is not known for sure what causes HG, but it has been thought to be associated with rapidly increasing human chorionic gonadotrophin (hCG) – a hormone that is secreted by the placenta as it forms early in pregnancy. Recent research has also suggested a link between HG and a growth-factor hormone called GDF15. Some pregnant people with HG produce abnormal levels of the hormone due to a variation in the gene code, but the research on this is still ongoing.

HG can sometimes improve as the pregnancy progresses, but some find no relief until the baby is born, even vomiting during labour. It can be a really lonely experience. Organisations such as Pregnancy Sickness Support were set up to support those affected so please do reach out to them if you're suffering from HG and it's impacting your mental and physical health.

FUEL FOR THE BUMP

Trying to consume anything other than beige foods, or even anything at all, might seem like quite an effort if you're in the throes of morning sickness, but keeping your body nourished is vital at this time, not only to help sustain your energy levels throughout your pregnancy, but to give your baby the nutrients they need to grow and develop. We've asked Dr Federica Amati to provide some guidance on how best to fuel yourself during each trimester and what to avoid, as well as answer the age-old question of whether we should actually be eating for two.

DIET, NUTRITION AND ALCOHOL DURING YOUR PREGNANCY

Dr Federica Amati, Nutritionist

The first trimester of pregnancy is when the fused sperm-and-egg cell becomes an embryo and then a foetus, and this process relies on the mother's health and nutrition before conception (see page 30) for a few things to happen: primarily, for a comfortable and welcoming endometrium (the lining of the womb where the placenta will form at about 10 weeks) to develop, where the early collection of cells that will create the embryo can dig in and implant. The uterus has special glands that release hormones, proteins and nutrients to support the early embryo before the placenta forms. At this stage, the embryo relies on a temporary structure called the yolk sac for energy, nutrients and oxygen, until the placenta later takes over these functions to support the growing baby.

The first 9 to 10 weeks of life: the embryonic stage sees the formation of the heart, the beginnings of the brain and the entire central nervous system, as well as the eyes, heart, limbs, ears and gut. All of this happens before a functional placenta allows for nutrient and gaseous exchange between the mother and the foetus. This initial period of development is very sensitive because so much essential building work is going on. Drinking alcohol or smoking at this time (and any other time during pregnancy) is strongly discouraged – both act as teratogens, which are chemicals that can cause major problems for the developing baby. Caffeine's effect depends on the amount you consume and the frequency, and whether you are an efficient caffeine metaboliser or not. Since there is a clear association between higher caffeine consumption (more than three cups of coffee per day) and some pregnancy complications, I personally recommend sticking to decaffeinated coffee during pregnancy. One cappuccino occasionally is unlikely to do any harm, but decaf coffee still has a lot of the benefits of regular coffee for our gut microbiome, so for me it's the safest option.

The most important thing in the first trimester is to find opportunities to eat nutrient-dense whole foods whenever morning sickness allows. Find the time of day when you are most likely to be able to stomach a meal and use that time to eat whole fruits and vegetables, eggs, oily fish, whole grains and legumes. For some women this might mean making a nutrient-packed smoothie with berries, frozen cauliflower, spinach, banana, nuts and seeds; for others, it might be a home-made fish pie. For me, it was scrambled eggs with smoked salmon on rye bread and lots of snack pots packed with Cheddar cheese, red grapes, cubed cucumber, apple and chopped celery.

For the second and third trimester, most women will be feeling better and less nauseous, which means there can be more focus on flavour and building really good nutrition for birth and beyond. Eating a variety of nutrient-dense foods that are also high in essential nutrients is easiest when consuming an omnivorous diet. If you follow a vegan diet, it is important to work with a health professional to make sure you are getting enough nutrients to support a healthy pregnancy. It is possible to do so, but it requires more time to prepare foods, and you may need additional supplementation for micronutrients that occur in higher concentrations in animal products, such as iron, vitamin B12, iodine and calcium.

The idea of 'eating for two' is a myth but one that has some biological grounding, as there is an increased energy requirement in the third trimester, but it does not amount to twice what you would normally need to eat. It's more like an additional snack per day, which will cover the extra energy and nutrients needed for the final 12 weeks. I prefer to switch the 'eating for two' idea to 'building your best mealtime buddy'. Developing babies can start to taste different flavours because they 'practise' by swallowing the amniotic fluid from the second trimester. Introducing bitter foods like broccoli, exposing your baby to allergens like gluten, peanuts and eggs, and starting to build their tiny palate is a fun way to think about eating for two during pregnancy.

There is no need to get the scales out and perfectly weigh out your meals. As with the time leading up to conception, eating a wide variety of foods (following the Mediterranean dietary principles of mostly whole plants, nuts and seeds, legumes and beans, whole grains, oily fish, extra virgin olive oil and occasional good-quality meat) is a great way to build healthy, nourishing plates.

Avoid processed meats and raw or undercooked meat, eggs or fish, as well as foods that are high in vitamin A (like liver) or mercury (like tuna), and raw or unpasteurised cheeses and milk – this will reduce the risk of food-borne illness and give you peace of mind. Pregnancy offers a wonderful opportunity to prioritise your health and wellbeing as you grow a new life.

Whichever way you end up birthing your baby, there will be some blood loss, so making sure you have good iron stores in your blood is important. Eating iron-rich foods including beans, lentils, eggs, fish and meat in the third trimester, and making sure you know your own iron-level status, are really key. Check with your doctor if you're not sure about your levels or if you have a history of anaemia.

The third trimester is also the time to look after your gut and vaginal microbiome! The trillions of microbes that make up these incredible ecosystems collaborate in the third trimester to change the composition of your vaginal microbiome, to prepare a microbial blueprint specifically for your baby to adopt (literally!) on its way out through the birth canal. A healthy vaginal microbiome helps to prevent premature birth and delivers the beginning of a baby's new gut microbiome if they are born vaginally. The vaginal microbiome doesn't like disruption and diversity – lactobacilli are the favourite type of microbe, and we can support them in a few ways: always wipe from front to back; do not wash your vaginal area and avoid using fragranced soaps or bath bombs; eat fermented foods like yoghurt, kefir and sauerkraut, which provide these friendly bugs; wear cotton underwear and avoid regularly wearing thongs or G-strings, which could cause microbes from your back passage to migrate to your vaginal area. Always see your doctor if you notice an unusual change in the smell, colour or amount of your vaginal fluids.

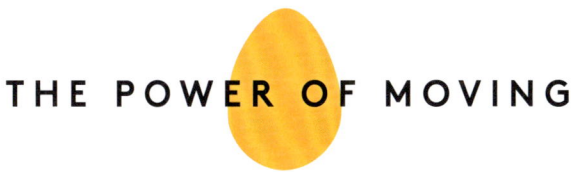

THE POWER OF MOVING

I know that nowadays I'm known for being the exercise lady, but I haven't always been like that. I actually only started training like I meant it when I was pregnant with my second daughter Tilly. I completely ballooned during my first pregnancy, so by the second I decided that I needed some kind of structured exercise routine in my life, which is when I started training with Jackie and Mark Wren. Some of you will know them from my workout DVDs – I made 15 DVDs, the majority with Jackie and Mark, and it was them who really inspired me to love exercise.

It will come as no surprise that I'm going to tell you that exercise is important at every stage of our lives, and pregnancy is no exception. In fact, keeping moving – or even starting to move – during your pregnancy will help you have a healthier, more comfortable experience, and exercises pose no risk to your baby. If you're someone who already exercises regularly, you can keep it up as long as you feel comfortable doing so and your doctor has okayed it. If you're doing fitness classes, make sure you let your instructor know that you're pregnant and how far along you are, so that they can modify necessary parts of the class for you.

If you're going to start exercising when you're pregnant, it's a good idea not to take on any vigorous, difficult or stressful new regime. Mark and Jackie put together a plan with a bit of strength training and some gentle cardio activity for me. This included things like speed walking (I live in the countryside so I would go for a brisk walk with Jackie) and weight-bearing exercises – lunges and arm work, for example.

If in doubt, just go for a walk. Walking is so underrated – it's brilliant for both your mental and physical health, and it's easy to build it into your life, so just shove on a pair of comfy shoes, maybe stick a podcast or some music in your ears and get outside.

If in doubt, just go for a walk.

5 (more) reasons to get moving during your pregnancy

EASE BACK PAIN

A growing bump puts extra pressure on your back, which can give you lower-back pain and make your pelvis ache. Strengthening your abdominal muscles can help counteract this, so speak to your midwife or a certified fitness instructor about dedicated pregnancy-safe exercises. Looking after your pelvic floor is a whole topic in itself, so I've asked Jenny Gillespie, who is a pelvic, obstetric and gynaecological physiotherapist, to tell you everything you need to know about that – turn to page 246 to find out what she has to say.

REDUCE THE RISK OF COMPLICATIONS

Exercise may reduce the likelihood of developing gestational diabetes (see page 146), which is a form of diabetes that affects at least 4–5 pregnant women out of 100 in the UK.[17] If you do develop it, moving your body will also help regulate your insulin levels.

SPEED UP YOUR RECOVERY POST-BIRTH

The fitter you are during pregnancy, the faster your body will recover physically after birth.

IMPROVE YOUR SLEEP

Getting a decent, restorative night's sleep can be a challenge when you're pregnant. Your boobs and bump get in the way, so you might just suffer bouts of insomnia because you can't get comfortable, and you might also be feeling anxious. Women who exercise say that they wake up feeling more rested than those who don't, so if you are having trouble sleeping, try getting some movement in during the day. I believe Mother Nature gives you restless sleep towards the end of your pregnancy, preparing you for life after birth.

SHORTEN YOUR LABOUR

Evidence now suggests that exercising during pregnancy could reduce the amount of time a woman spends in labour. Researchers at the Technical University of Madrid found that a supervised exercise programme during pregnancy decreased the duration of the first phase of labour as well as the total labour time. As somebody who was in labour for 36 hours with Holly, I can tell you that any incentive to shorten it would have been right up my street.

YOUR STORIES

'They say there are two types of expecting mothers: those who go with the flow and those who do the research.' — Aisling

I felt like I was doing a PhD in 'birthing'. I read books on labour and pregnancy, completed online courses and spoke with mothers who had gone before me. I stayed active, still weight training until the day before I went into labour, and I worked with the incredible midwives to develop a birth plan. I was lucky enough to have a vaginal birth with no medical intervention or pain relief. It was the most incredible experience of my life, and I have never felt so strong, physically, mentally and emotionally. Women are superhuman.

Davina: I totally agree, Aisling – it's amazing what women's bodies can do and how much strength we have. I've never felt as much respect for my body and its abilities as during pregnancy and birth – it's made me want to look after mine and acknowledge all the work it's done as I've got older.

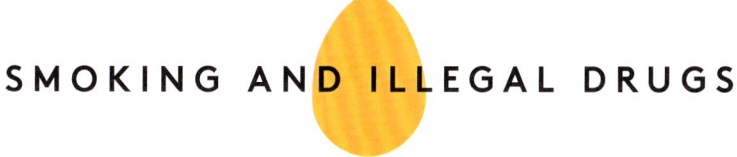

SMOKING AND ILLEGAL DRUGS

As a former addict, I really do understand that, like all addictions, smoking can be a very hard habit to kick, but there are over 4,000 chemicals in each cigarette and these can be very harmful to your baby, so if ever there was a time to try to quit, it is now. Stopping smoking or vaping during your pregnancy will help increase your chances of having a healthy baby and will reduce the risk of complications during your labour and of having a stillbirth. Passive smoke can also harm your growing baby, so do speak to anybody in your household who smokes.

Drugs are a complicated one because while street drugs can cross the placenta and affect your baby and its organs while it is growing, coming off drugs suddenly can also be dangerous for you and your baby. I know it might feel shameful or difficult, but if it affects you, try to talk to your midwife or doctor about your drug use so that you can get the support you need.

FEELING VULNERABLE AND DEFENDING THE BUMP

I want to talk about vulnerability during pregnancy, because I think, as a society, it's something we need to be very aware of. In fact, I think we need to reframe the way we treat and speak to pregnant women. There is something about carrying a baby in your tummy that makes you very conscious of the way you are treated. A survival instinct kicks in and you start to think, I've got to really take care of myself and this baby, making you want to feel calm and safe at all times.

Having said that, I was presenting *Big Brother* throughout all three of my pregnancies and, weirdly, I actually loved the chaos of it. It was noisy and shouty, but it felt so exciting. I just loved that job so much, and I think the babies could sense that and felt soothed by it, because they always fell asleep when I was presenting. And yet I remember going to watch a *Star Wars* movie when I was pregnant and the noise in the cinema was so loud that I wanted to put three coats over my tummy to protect it. That bump makes you feel vulnerable – you are already mothering this little being in your tummy and you will do anything to protect them – so I feel very strongly that we need to do our utmost to make sure we in turn protect pregnant women and help them feel safe, calm and cared for whenever we're around them.

And to any partners reading this book, please do try to protect your pregnant partner from negativity around childbirth as you support her on this journey: learn, teach others, use calming language and avoid people who might fire her up or worry her in any way.

Another thing I would like you to do when you're pregnant is to feel empowered to tell people if you would rather they didn't touch your bump. There is something very inviting about a pregnant belly, and very often people feel extremely confident in reaching out to touch or massage it. For many of you that will be absolutely fine. I didn't generally mind it, but there were a couple of occasions when it made me feel very uncomfortable, and lots of you will also find it very invasive. So I think it's helpful to come up with a sentence that you can use every time somebody goes towards your belly if you don't want them to touch it. It could be something like: 'I'm so sorry, I'm a bit funny about anyone touching my belly.' Or, 'I hope you don't mind but I'd rather you didn't touch my bump.' Or you can find a really gentle excuse like, 'Would you mind not touching my bump? The baby is resting at the moment and I don't want it to start kicking again.'

You become a mother from the minute you conceive, and even when people can't see your pregnancy, it doesn't mean that you feel any less protective of your growing baby.

CONFLICTING EVIDENCE AND VOICES

One of the things I found hardest when I was pregnant was how many different voices there were offering advice and how many of those voices were telling me things I didn't want to hear or what I was doing was wrong. I felt as though I'd completely lost my voice. In her book *Spiritual Midwifery*, Ina May Gaskin talks about tuning in to our 'monkey', which is basically our intuition and primal instinct as a pregnant woman. We know that women have been giving birth for millennia, so we simply need to trust ourselves and our instincts. With your first birth especially, you're very susceptible to other people's opinions, but my advice is to think hard about what feels right to YOU – you will KNOW when something feels off-kilter, particularly when it comes to labour. Ask yourself: do I want to be lying down? Do I want to be standing up? What's my body telling me? I knew when I wanted to get out of bed to start walking around to get the baby in the right position. It just felt right, so I knew, I've got to walk. Listen to yourself, trust yourself. And if you need to ask people for advice, ask medical professionals around you who really know what they're talking about.

And while this book is all about encouraging women to speak out and get their voices heard, tragically in the UK there are still communities of women who aren't being listened to, let alone being taken into account.

I met Tinuke Awe and Clo Abe at a talk they were giving about Black maternity, and was struck by how eloquent and what great communicators they were. Tinuke and Clo are the founders of Five X More, an organisation whose mission is to empower, support and advocate for Black women in childbirth, ensuring they receive the respectful, equitable, and high-quality care they deserve during pregnancy and beyond.

When I met them, they explained some of the gaping differences there are between Black and white women's experience of maternity in the UK, and as they outline over the page, the statistics around Black maternal deaths during pregnancy are shocking – today Black women in the UK are 2.9 times more likely to die during pregnancy than white women (it was 5 times more but their amazing work has changed that). Tinuke and Clo use their platform to campaign for parity, to lobby government and make recommendations to the NHS. They are powerhouses – women who get shit done –and it's an honour to have them in this book to tell their story and outline the work Five X More does and the changes they are seeing happen as a result.

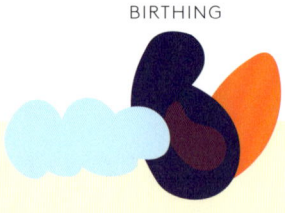

BLACK MATERNITY

FIVE X MORE

Black women in the UK are 2.9 times[18] more likely to die in pregnancy, childbirth and the six-week postpartum period in comparison to white women. Historically this figure was five times more.[19] Let's take you on a little journey through time to understand a bit more about how we got here.

Dr James Marion Sims (1813–1883), the 'father of modern gynaecology',[20] is the creator of the Sims Speculum, which is a gynaecological instrument that is still used in modern medicine. Sims was praised for his revolutionary approach to treating the diseases of women but many people are unaware of the shocking practices he performed on enslaved Black women while he was perfecting this instrument.

Dr Sims performed these inhumane operations without anaesthesia under the misguided belief that Black people did not feel pain. When the instrument was perfected he used it on white women under anaesthesia.

Dr Sims was celebrated for his medical achievements; however, his false beliefs about Black people's inability to feel pain have continued to live on to this day.

In 2015, a nursing textbook published by Pearson made a controversial claim about Black people, stating that they 'often report higher pain intensity than other cultures' and believe 'suffering and pain are inevitable'.[21] This statement sparked significant backlash and criticism for perpetuating harmful stereotypes and following widespread condemnation on social media, the textbook was pulled from circulation in 2017.

A 2016 study showed that white medical students and soon-to-be doctors held incorrect unconscious biases about Black people, believing they 'had thicker skin' and 'fewer nerve endings'.[22] They also attributed higher pain tolerance to Black patients and were less likely to administer pain relief to them.

Further evidence of systemic prejudice in healthcare emerged from a 2022 survey conducted by the Black Equity Organisation, which revealed that 65 per cent of Black respondents had

My experience was tainted with feelings of not being listened to and believed when I said I was in labour and I eventually had to have a ventouse delivery.

experienced prejudice from healthcare professionals.[23] This figure increased to 75 per cent among Black individuals aged 18 to 34.

In 2017, I (Tinuke) had a terrible experience of giving birth to my son. I had pre-eclampsia that was diagnosed very late in my pregnancy and it led me to be induced. My experience was tainted with feelings of not being listened to and believed when I said I was in labour and I eventually had to have a ventouse delivery. I feel like it would have been avoided if I had simply been listened to in the first place. I remember feeling like I didn't matter, that my voice was not important. I was just grateful that my baby was okay.

I have a platform called Mums and Tea where I host events for mothers. That's where I found out my birthing experience was not an isolated one as many women on the platform also had negative experiences. It was heartbreaking to hear.

In 2018 the MBRRACE-UK report (Mothers and Babies: Reducing Risk through Audits and Confidential Enquiries across the UK)[24] statistics stated that at that time Black women were 5 times more likely to die in pregnancy, childbirth and the 6-week postpartum period compared to white women. I wanted to do something about it so I contacted Clo who was working in perinatal mental health at the time for us to host a one off event to highlight these stats. We ended up building Five X More.

After doing a deeper dive into the research we were shocked at what we found in relation to the disparities.

Reports dating back to 1994[25] indicated that the risk of maternal death might be higher in Black women. However, specific data on ethnicity was not collected at the time, preventing precise figures. By 1998, it was documented that Black women had a three times greater risk of maternal mortality compared to their white counterparts and over the years the dial has not moved and the statistics are still poorer for Black women.

We often get asked why this disparity exists. What we do know from the statistics is that Black women are dying from the same things as white women, just at a significantly higher rate. There are multiple reasons as to why this happens, from healthcare professionals not knowing what certain conditions look like on darker skin thanks to the current medical curriculum, to the myths and stereotypes such as Black women having 'African pelvises' making it difficult to give birth.[26]

Over the years we have seen significant changes in the maternity space, including the commencement of the government's maternity disparities taskforce, the race disparities taskforce from the Royal College of Obstetricians and Gynaecologists (RCOG), the NHS Race and Health Observatory and many instances of Black maternal health being featured in the news and in notable publications in order to raise awareness.

At Five X More, we aim to create real long-lasting change by empowering Black women with knowledge and resources, helping them feel in control of their birthing experiences. Through our lobbying efforts, there was a historic debate[27] in Parliament on Black Maternal Healthcare and Mortality in 2021, driven by our petition that garnered over 187,000 signatures.

Despite this, the debate did not lead to a focused initiative on reducing Black maternal deaths. It did, however, play a huge part in raising awareness and reaching a wider audience. To push for more substantial action, we launched a survey on Black women's maternity experiences, similar to MBRRACE-UK but exclusively for our community. This survey and subsequent report[28] aimed to shed light on their unique challenges and advocate for tailored healthcare improvements and is the largest survey on Black maternity experiences in the UK so far. It must be noted that Black women and birthing people are diverse, with varied thoughts and experiences, and we do not represent all Black women.

The key takeaways from the survey include:

— Black women do actually participate in research.

— Respondents generally earned above the national average, were degree-educated and were married or in relationships.

— Black women complained less than Black mixed women, despite receiving poorer care.

From our survey, women expressed the following needs for improving maternity services:

— Health professionals should avoid making assumptions based on ethnicity.

— Women want to be listened to and heard.

— Women want to be told about all their birthing options.

We are proud of the work we are doing with Five X More but we wish we didn't exist. What we hope for is that in the future we are no longer having the same conversations about Black Women dying and that the disparities no longer exist. We also hope that women's health in general is a top priority and is taken more seriously.

If you would like to support us, follow us on our social media platforms, write to your local MP to find out what they are doing in their local constituencies to help decrease the disparities and in general, continue to have these important discussions. You can't change something you don't know about.

By 1998, it was documented that Black women had a three times greater risk of maternal mortality compared to their white counterparts.

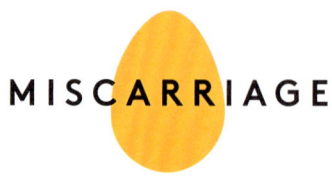

MISCARRIAGE

I have friends who have lost babies through miscarriages and friends who have had stillbirths, and I cannot imagine the excruciating pain they have been through. Miscarriage affects 10 to 20 per cent of first-trimester pregnancies, and 1 to 2 per cent of second-trimester pregnancies,[29] with the risk increasing with age,[30] which is why it is such an important topic to address. Through each of my pregnancies I fully acknowledged to myself that sometimes babies don't make it and I think it's good to have that in the back of our minds.

A miscarriage is the loss of a baby before they can survive outside the uterus and is legally defined as the loss of a baby in the uterus before 24 weeks' gestation. Occasionally babies are born alive before 24 weeks, but the majority will unfortunately not survive. If this happens, it's referred to as a neonatal death. Opposite, Marley has outlined some possible causes of miscarriage to help you understand why they happen.

It's also important to know the symptoms. Possibly, you'd be in pain with cramps, or have vaginal bleeding (which can range from light spotting to heavy bleeding). You might pass tissue or clots, and will also notice that you've stopped experiencing pregnancy symptoms, such as tender breasts and nausea. Sometimes there are no obvious physical signs, and it will only be discovered when you go for an ultrasound. You do also

need to know that light bleeding or spotting is relatively common in the first trimester and doesn't necessarily mean you're having a miscarriage, so if you start bleeding, contact your midwife and check with them. If you're less than six weeks pregnant your midwife may suggest you wait, or, depending on how far along the pregnancy is, you'll be referred to an early pregnancy unit, or maternity unit.

Usually, a miscarriage will pass out in one or two weeks, but sometimes you might have to take medicine to help with that. If your miscarriage is discovered on an ultrasound, you can ask to have a procedure known as a dilation and curettage (D&C) to remove matter from the uterus.

The most heartbreaking thing is that from the moment you are pregnant you love your baby and consider it part of your family. I have friends who often talk about the child they lost and they always remain a family member.

Your midwife or maternity team can offer you support and guidance. They can provide information about what to expect physically and emotionally, answer any questions you may have and offer options for follow-up care for future pregnancies. They can also connect you with additional resources, such as counsellors or support groups, to help you. Tommy's charity and the Miscarriage Association are organisations that support people who have experienced miscarriage. You can try for another baby as soon as your symptoms have passed, and you feel ready. If this is happening to you now, I'm sending you so much love.

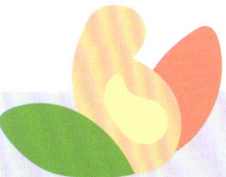

WHY DO MISCARRIAGES HAPPEN?

Midwife Marley

A miscarriage can be devastating. It is a common and heartbreaking experience, and the true rate of incidence may be even higher than we know, since many miscarriages happen very early in pregnancy before a woman realises she is pregnant.

Although miscarriage is a traumatic experience at any stage, late miscarriages in the second trimester can be particularly difficult to navigate. Foetal movements may have been felt, the 'baby bump' may be visible and the mother will likely experience a labour, giving birth to the baby. Late miscarriages often happen at a time when the pregnancy has been announced to friends and family, which can add another layer of difficulty when breaking the sad news.

If someone suffers from multiple miscarriages (three or more), they may be referred to an obstetric doctor for tests to help identify why recurrent losses are occurring. Often, it's impossible to understand why a miscarriage has occurred, but there are some potential contributing factors:

— **Chromosomal Abnormalities:** It is thought that a high number of miscarriages, particularly first-trimester miscarriages, occur due to genetic or chromosomal abnormalities in the embryo, which prevent it from developing normally.

— **Maternal Health Factors:** Certain maternal health conditions, such as diabetes, thyroid disorders, autoimmune diseases and infections, can increase the risk of miscarriage.

— **Uterine or Cervical Issues:** Structural abnormalities in the uterus or cervix, such as fibroids or cervical weakness, can contribute to miscarriage.

— **Lifestyle Factors:** Smoking, excessive alcohol consumption, drug use and exposure to environmental toxins can increase the risk of miscarriage.

— **Advanced Maternal Age:** Women over the age of 35 are at higher risk of miscarriage due to age-related decline in egg quality.

— **Hormonal Imbalances:** If there is an imbalance in the hormones crucial for maintaining pregnancy, such as progesterone, this can lead to miscarriage.

Early miscarriages up to 12 weeks' gestation can occur in different ways:

— An ectopic pregnancy, which develops outside the uterus (i.e. in the fallopian tubes) and isn't able to develop properly.

— Placenta Previa: When the placenta implants too low in the uterus it can obstruct the birth canal and cause miscarriage, especially in the early stages.

— A chemical pregnancy, in which the egg is fertilised but doesn't implant properly in the womb. This can mean a positive pregnancy test is produced but no foetal sac is identified in an ultrasound.

— A blighted ovum, in which the fertilised egg implants in the lining of the uterus but only forms a placenta and not an embryo.

— A pregnancy that develops initially as it should but, for unknown reasons, miscarries spontaneously.

Coping with miscarriage is a deeply personal process, and there's no right or wrong way to grieve. If you experience a miscarriage, whether you are a mother or father, it's essential to allow yourself to feel your emotions and seek support from loved ones, support groups or mental health professionals if needed, when you are ready.

Up until recently, babies lost before 24 weeks were not recognised legally – there was no death certificate that formally recognised the baby. But in early 2024, the UK Government decided to begin issuing formal baby-loss certificates to those who have experienced the early loss of their baby. This has been welcomed by many campaigners and parents who have experienced the trauma.

For information about where to go for support and guidance if you experience miscarriage, please see page 309.

'It was our first pregnancy and my husband and I were so excited.' — Beth

I was nervous when I found out I was pregnant, but I also felt ready, like something had shifted in my mindset, and I truly wanted to be a mother.

The first 12 weeks had been smooth and we walked into our 12-week scan without a second thought that anything could be wrong. I remember lying on the bed, watching the sonographer move the ultrasound probe across my belly.

She was quiet for a long time and kept pressing down. The clock on the wall was a NICE DAY clock and I remember thinking something was wrong. That this wasn't going to be a nice day at all.

Then she spoke.

'I think there's a problem. I can't find the heartbeat.'

Everything after that is a blur. I remember screaming. Crying. Being led to a small, grey room where a doctor gently explained what would happen next. A few days later, I had the operation. And just like that, the pregnancy was over.

I cannot put into words how heartbreaking it was. Life moves on, and we got through it, but even now, I feel a sadness for the people we were – the ones who walked into that scan full of hope, never imagining how lost we were about to feel.

Davina: Beth, I don't even know what to say, except thank you. Your story will help other people going through something similar. I think we can all turn up at the 12-week scan thinking, *I've got to three months without a miscarriage; everything must be fine,* so it is important for us to know that that is not always the case.

I am so sorry this happened to you both, and I'm just sending you lots of love and enormous gratitude for sharing your story with us.

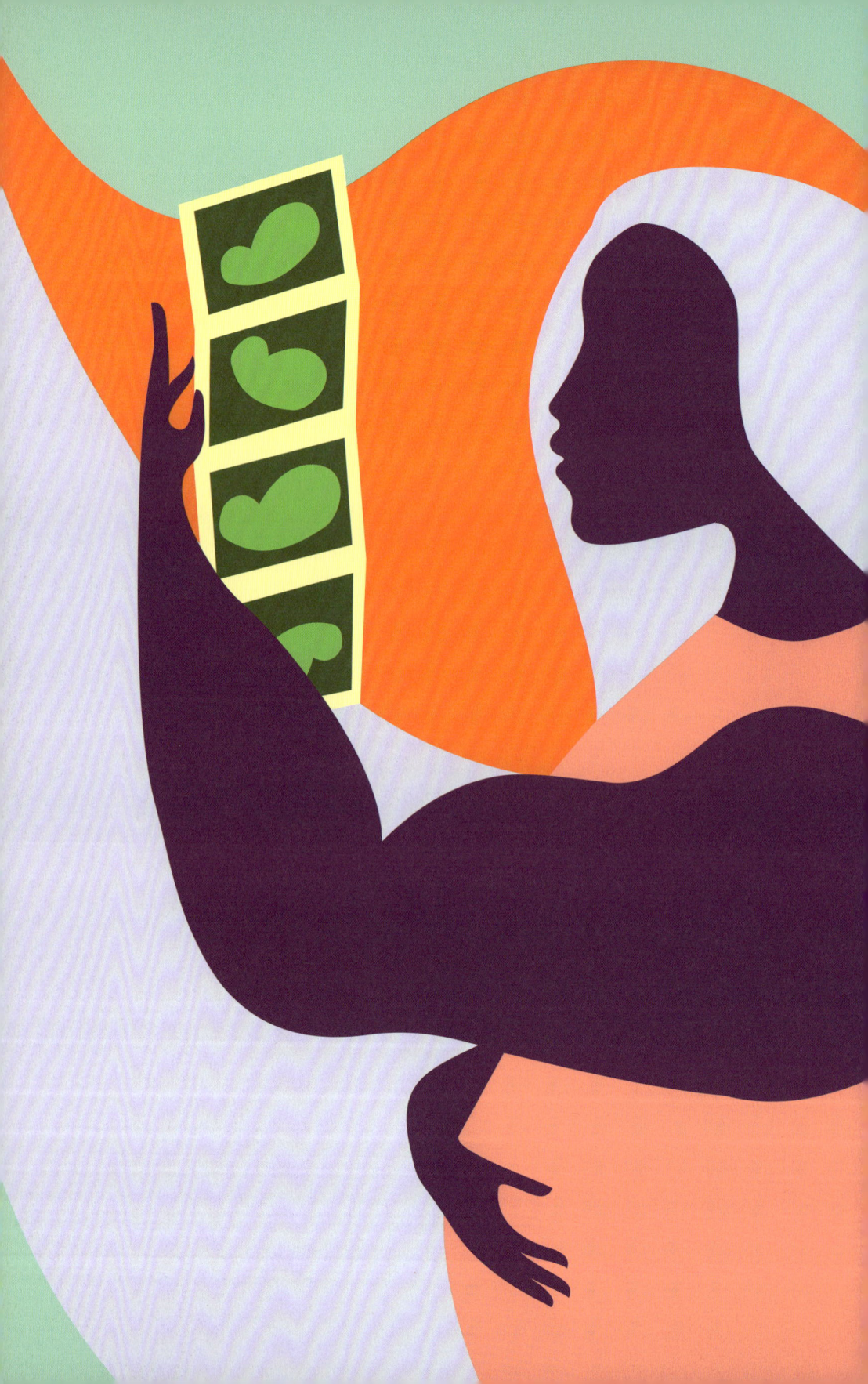

CHAPTER 3

SECOND TRIMESTER

13–27 WEEKS

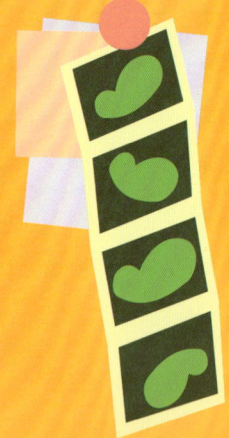

A lot of women start to feel as if their pregnancy is more 'real' at this stage.

CHANGE IS COMING

You'll have had your first scan, your bump might be showing, and if your first scan went well and there aren't any concerns about the viability of your pregnancy, you might be starting to tell people you're having a baby. That brings with it a lot of change. You have to start confronting and preparing for this next stage in your life, and your new identity and role, and that can feel daunting, so I'll talk a bit in this chapter about what that shifting identity means and how to navigate it, as I think lots of us fail to realise that amid all the excitement, there is also quite a bit of fear and nervousness about the loss of our pre-pregnant self. Where have I gone?

Also, my morning sickness suddenly stopped a few weeks into this trimester, which was such a relief, and for lots of women that's the case (but it can also be a bit of a worry, so if you are worried, talk to your midwife). Hopefully you'll be feeling a bit less queasy, although pregnancy does tend to come with a whole host of other joys, including swollen ankles and headaches, among others, so we've outlined what might be ahead physically, too.

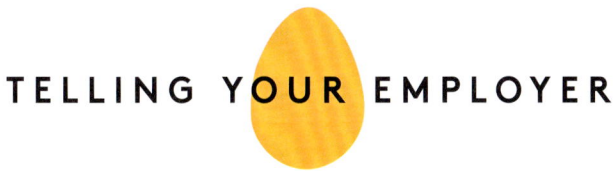

TELLING YOUR EMPLOYER

While you might want to shout it from the rooftops and tell anyone who will listen that you're pregnant, telling your employer could be a different story. Lots of you have shared with me that it can be quite nerve-racking talking to your boss – you were worried about how they were going to react or whether pregnancy was going to have implications for your career. So, I just want to get a bit shouty for a moment and remind anyone who has yet speak to their employer: the fact that you are choosing to become a parent, and that biologically you are obliged to be the one carrying this baby, should have ABSOLUTELY NO IMPACT on your career. However, it's still a really good idea to check what the laws are around your rights when taking maternity or paternity leave so that you understand them fully. We've included details in the resources section on page 313.

Most people wait until they are around 12 weeks pregnant to tell their workplace, mainly because they are holding off until the 12-week dating scan to check that the baby is healthy and the pregnancy is progressing smoothly. However, if you are experiencing really bad morning sickness, I think you owe it to yourself to let your boss know sooner than that, which means you might have to tell them quite early on in your pregnancy. If you're spending hours in the loo being sick or are looking pretty peaky, it can be difficult to hide it, and you might need support from your employer if you're having to rest a lot and need some time off work because you are feeling so ill.

Generally speaking, you might not want too many people at work knowing you're pregnant. I was someone that told quite a lot of people I loved because I knew that if I did miscarry, I would need their support. Choose carefully is what I'm saying. Legally, you don't have to tell your employer until 15 weeks before your due date (essentially at 25 weeks), especially if you would like to go back to your job at some point after the birth and want to be eligible for statutory maternity pay. If you do want to take maternity leave or claim maternity pay then you need to advise your employer about your pregnancy in writing. You can also have paid time off for antenatal care, appointments and some antenatal classes, which is another reason to tell your boss as soon as you feel you can. Partners are also entitled to time off for two antenatal appointments, though they're unpaid.

If you're worried about the chat with your boss, the best thing you can do is arm yourself with all the information and your answers to any questions that might come up. Knowledge is power, so do your research and think about the things you'd like to discuss and agree with your boss. Here are some tips to help you prepare for the conversation:

— Have a look at your employment contract and your organisation's pregnancy and maternity policy.

— Check the most up-to-date information on the GOV.UK website to find out about your legal entitlements, such as statutory maternity leave, keeping-in-touch (KIT) days and shared parental leave.

— Your doctor or midwife will give you a MAT B1 form after your 20-week scan. This is proof of pregnancy and the estimated week of birth, which is essential for claiming maternity pay and leave. Give it to your employer when applying for Statutory Maternity Pay (SMP) or to the government when applying for Maternity Allowance.

— Think about dates that might be relevant to your boss at this point: antenatal appointments, your due date and any holiday you'd like to take (you'll also eventually need to think about when you'd like to start your maternity leave).

The prospect of stopping work for a time and having a reduced income is likely to feel quite daunting. But as with so much of this journey, there are ways to manage your finances. Planning for what's to come will help remove some of the anxiety and allow you to feel in control. To help you understand and calculate the financial implications of having a baby, we've asked Emilie Bellet, founder of the online financial community for women Vestpod, to talk you through how to plan and budget for the next few months and beyond.

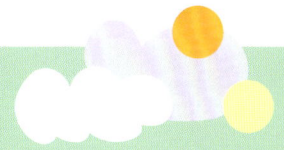

BABIES AND BUDGETS: FINANCIAL REALITIES BEYOND THE BASICS

Emilie Bellet, Founder of Vestpod

Becoming a parent involves more than just budgeting for prams and nappies. While many expect the basic costs, it's often the unexpected financial challenges that cause the most stress. From navigating childcare costs to understanding maternity pay, here's how to approach pregnancy and parenthood with a solid financial plan.

1. UNDERSTANDING MATERNITY PAY: MORE THAN JUST STATUTORY MATERNITY PAY (SMP)

Many new mums rely on Statutory Maternity Pay (SMP), but the reality is that it's often less than you expect – 90 per cent of your average weekly earnings (before tax) for the first six weeks and the statutory maternity pay or 90 per cent of your average weekly earnings (whichever is lower) for the next 33 weeks. This drop can be a financial shock for low-income or self-employed women. Employers may offer enhanced maternity packages, so it's essential to check your options.

Tip: Speak with your HR team about enhanced benefits, or check your eligibility for Maternity Allowance if you're self-employed. Budget around SMP to see how your household will manage and save where necessary.

2. MEDICAL COSTS: WHAT'S FREE AND WHAT'S NOT

The NHS offers great maternity care, but not all is free. Expect costs for prescriptions, dental work beyond free care, and possibly extra scans. Unexpected post-birth costs like physiotherapy or a lactation consultant can also arise.

Tip: Apply for your maternity exemption certificate for free prescriptions and dental care. Set aside funds for any private healthcare needs like antenatal classes or specialist care.

3. PARENTAL LEAVE FOR PARTNERS

Shared parental leave in the UK allows up to 50 weeks of leave between both parents, but statutory pay is similar to SMP, which could lead to a significant drop in income if both parents take time off.

Tip: Plan early for how you'll share leave and manage financial gaps. Ask your partner's employer about enhanced parental pay and make informed decisions on leave sharing.

4. CHILDCARE: START PLANNING SOONER THAN YOU THINK

Childcare in the UK can cost more than £1,000 a month (although costs can vary significantly across regions), especially for full-time nursery care. However, paying for childcare can be seen as an investment in maintaining your career and future earnings.

Tip: Start researching childcare options (such as a child minder, nanny or nursery) early and take advantage of government schemes like Tax-Free Childcare or free childcare hours. Keep in mind that waiting lists can be long, so plan ahead.

5. THE MOTHERHOOD PENALTY: PROTECTING YOUR CAREER AND INCOME

The 'motherhood penalty' is the economic hit women often take at work after becoming mothers. Unlike men, who sometimes get a 'fatherhood bonus', women's earnings can drop by up to 30 per cent after having children. This happens because of several factors: time off, working fewer hours, or simply being passed over for promotions or high-profile projects due to assumptions about their availability. Over time, this impact on pay and career growth widens the gender pay gap and can affect long-term financial security.

Tip: Before going on leave, talk to your employer about maintaining your career progression. Consider upskilling or carrying out smaller projects during maternity leave.

6. THE SILENT HIT TO YOUR RETIREMENT

Maternity leave or working reduced hours can lead to gaps in pension contributions, which can affect your retirement savings.

Tip: If possible, make voluntary National Insurance contributions to fill

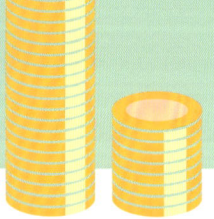

any gaps and try to keep your pension contributions consistent to avoid long-term impacts. Your partner could also increase their contributions or make contributions on your behalf to keep your savings on track.

7. PREPARING FOR THE UNEXPECTED

Once you have a child, unexpected expenses multiply – whether it's unplanned doctor visits or replacing outgrown clothes. Having a solid emergency fund is key.

Tip: Sit down with your partner to discuss how you'll manage new financial pressures. Agree on a savings goal to cover at least three to six months of expenses and decide how to handle sudden costs when they arise.

8. NAVIGATING GOVERNMENT SUPPORT

New parents can access various support schemes, but they aren't always well known. Child Benefit is available to all parents, though it may be taxed back if one partner earns more than £60,000. Universal Credit is available for low-income families, and the NHS Healthy Start scheme provides free vitamins, milk and food vouchers for eligible families.

Tip: Use online benefit calculators from Turn2Us or the Government website to check your eligibility for Child Benefit, Universal Credit or the Healthy Start scheme.

9. PLANNING FOR UNEXPECTED WORK CHANGES

If you're employed, your working hours may not look the same post-maternity leave. Some parents find full-time work no longer viable due to childcare costs, while others seek flexible or part-time work.

If you're not currently working and are in a relationship, there's still support available to help secure your financial future. Taking small steps like setting up a budget with a partner or looking into ISAs and partner pension contributions can help build long-term financial security.

Tip: If you're currently employed, explore flexible working options with your employer before going on leave. For those considering part-time work upon return, think about how this may affect not only your immediate income, but also long-term goals like pensions and career growth. And if you're not working, look into support options like Universal Credit, Child Benefit and partner pension contributions.

10. BUDGETING TIPS FOR SOLO MUMS: BUILDING FINANCIAL SECURITY

Managing finances solo requires careful planning to cover essentials, unexpected costs and future savings.

Tip: Track your monthly expenses, focusing on essentials like rent, childcare and groceries. Set up an automatic transfer to a savings account each payday, even if it's a small amount – over time, it adds up. To handle larger expenses, such as school uniforms or childcare, plan ahead by setting aside a little each month, which can ease the financial impact when these costs arise.

11. A HEAD START FOR YOUR CHILD'S FUTURE

Though it may seem far off, starting to save for your child's future can reduce financial burdens later. Consider opening a Junior ISA for tax-free growth or a children's pension. Navigating the school system can be daunting, so research your options early.

Think of this time as your opportunity to take control and tackle money challenges head-on. Build your safety net, invest in your future and create a financial game plan that sets you up for success. Enjoy the journey!

Approaching pregnancy and parenthood with a solid financial plan is the first step to feeling more in control.

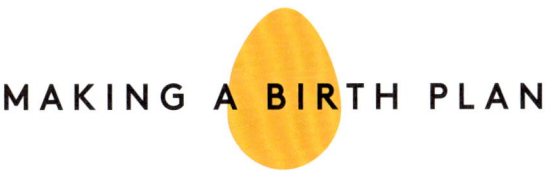

MAKING A BIRTH PLAN

The reason I'm so passionate about the subject of giving birth is that I want you to have the best chance of experiencing a positive birth – a birth that is right for you, your baby and your partner. And for me, the starting point for that is to make a birth plan.

Essentially, a birth plan is a formal record of what you would like to happen during your labour. It details as much or as little as you'd like, but it can specify everything from where you want to give birth and who will be with you, to which pain relief you want to use, how and whether you would like your baby's heart rate monitored during the birth and whether you want the baby lifted onto you for skin-to-skin contact before the cord is cut.

You don't have to create a plan, but my experience – and the fact that I completely changed my birth plan in the second trimester of my first pregnancy to give birth at home – convinced me that it's really helpful to have one at this stage, as it lets your birthing partner and the medical professionals working with you know your wishes and preferences. Because, believe me, once you go into labour, you will not want to be making any big decisions about the kind of birth you want. And if anybody else is trying to make decisions during your labour that don't reflect what you had in mind, you're just not going to have the strength to put your point forward.

And, as I discovered with Caroline, talking your birth plan through with your midwife gives them a chance to get to know you, which means that they'll have a better understanding of what you're hoping to achieve, and therefore what direction things should go in if your plans need to change.

This section is about arming you with the facts I wish I'd had before I got 20 weeks down the road, so that you have the knowledge to make informed decisions about every aspect of your birth, and are able to write your birth plan and explain to your midwife, your partner or birthing partner, and the doctors what YOU want and what YOU need. Read, study and absorb Chapter 5: BIRTH (see page 162), as that will help give you an overview of everything else you may encounter during birth and need to think about.

In terms of writing the plan itself, there are different ways you can do this. Your midwife or hospital might have a template to give you, or if you have a look at the 'Labour and birth' section on the NHS website, they've got a really brilliant template, which takes you through all the things you need to consider (don't worry if you're not sure about your choices for everything at this stage – there's still time to make those decisions). If you're writing your own, just make sure it's legible and simple to follow – the midwife you see in hospital won't necessarily be familiar with you or your plan, so you want to make sure it's really clear for them to follow. Marley's given you some extra pointers on how to write the plan itself (see page 100), and over the next few pages are the things you need to consider.

CHOOSING WHERE TO GIVE BIRTH

Thinking about where you want to give birth is the number-one decision to make, because wherever you are, you want to feel comfortable and safe. I think it's something you want to start thinking about within the first few weeks of your pregnancy. That doesn't mean you can't change your mind – when I made the decision to give birth at home, I had already been booked in to give birth in hospital – but it's useful to gather the information early on. I loved talking to anybody who had recently had a baby – I wanted to hear about all the different ways you could give birth, from the perspective of those who'd done it, so that's a great place to start, but if you don't have friends who have started having babies yet, you could talk to relatives, work colleagues or, of course, your midwife. It was through chatting to my friend Annabel, who'd given birth at home, that I realised I needed to get hold of all the information I could and consider each option from every angle before my husband and I made the decision about the kind of birth we wanted to have and where we wanted it to be. Because if you are on this journey with a partner, your birth plan is something you should discuss with them so that they feel involved and part of the decision-making process.

Essentially, if you are having your baby in the UK, you have three options for where to give birth:

1 **At home**

2 **In a midwifery unit (also called birth centres)**

3 **In hospital**

If your birth is being managed through the NHS, the option you go for will be influenced by your needs and risks, but also partly by where you live, because not every hospital has a birth centre, nor do they necessarily have enough midwives to be able to send them to your home at the time you give birth. Your midwife will be able to discuss the options in your area.

You can also travel outside of your NHS Trust's area, but please bear in mind that if your labour develops very fast, that's going to add stress and pressure to the experience. As well as from your midwife, you can get information about the different options available to you from your GP, local maternity unit and also through maternity and neonatal voices partnerships (MNVPs). MNVPs are NHS local working groups made up of women and their families, midwives, doctors and other health professionals, all joining forces to plan, review and contribute to the development of local maternity care. They are independently led and ensure that service-user voices are at the heart of decision-making in maternity and neonatal services. Each MNVP is led by someone who is both independent (not otherwise employed by the NHS) and lay (not trained as a doctor, nurse or midwife).

If you've got a medical condition, the advice is to give birth in hospital where you've got specialists around you in case you need any kind of treatment, as this is safest, but if you're healthy and have no complications and aren't restricted by your area, you can choose any of these locations.

HOME BIRTH

When I spoke to my midwives about home birth, they asked me loads of questions about my health, they asked me for my medical history, took my blood pressure – I mean, they really gave me a proper once-over. And they said (because I was asking them about it) that, for me, home birth could be an option.

If you're having your first baby, home birth does slightly increase the risk of problems for the baby: 9 in 1,000 babies die in a home birth, whereas 5 in 1,000 babies die in a hospital birth,[31] so that is something you need to take into account. But if you're having your second or third baby, a planned home birth is as safe as having your baby in hospital or a midwife-led unit.

Here are the things you need to consider when thinking about a home birth:

— You don't have specialist care at home – you're going to be with a midwife, and usually two midwives, which is wonderful, but you won't have big bits of equipment there, so

if you need them, you're going to have to be transferred to a hospital.

— You're also not going to be able to have an epidural – you can have other forms of pain relief, but you are going to have to experience pain of some kind at some point.

However, there are also some advantages to giving birth at home:

— You're going to feel much more relaxed, which is largely why I wanted to do it; I felt much safer knowing I was in my own surroundings.

— The midwives had told me that there was a lower likelihood of having interventions such as forceps (see page 207) or a ventouse (also page 207) or an episiotomy (see page 195) at home, and I was keen to avoid them, so that was another driver for me.

— Sometimes, though not in all cases, it will mean that you can give birth with a midwife with whom you've built up a relationship. They are often the person you will have seen at the birth centre or the hospital, and they will be the person who comes out to deliver your baby. And that's really nice.

— I loved all the familiarity that comes with being at home: eating food from your kitchen, being in your sheets, having all your own things around you. All that just made it feel very comforting; I knew I was in a safe, nurturing place.

— It is a calm and private environment where you can start your new life with your baby without being watched by lots of strangers and without the noise and bustle of a busy postnatal ward.

— When I had my second and third babies, I loved having my other kids around me. I've got some great pictures of Holly from that time – I was in a birthing pool and she was desperate to get in with me. I had to tell her that was NOT a good idea! She was so into helping me through each contraction. And then, when I transitioned (the shift from the first stage of labour to the second stage – see page 176) and I had a little cry, she got me a tissue. It was the sweetest thing. Having my older kids around helped me be brave, but I also felt like I wanted them to see and realise that giving birth is a powerful moment for a woman.

If you are thinking of a home birth, but you're a bit nervous about it, know that you can change your mind, even on the day. I didn't decide for definite that I was going to have a home birth until I was halfway through my labour. In the early stages I said to Pam, 'I'm not sure I'm going to want to have the baby at home, I might be a bit nervous.' And she said, 'I'm going to tell the hospital now that you are in labour, then, at a certain point in your labour, I'm going to tell you that now is the time that we should go to a hospital if you want to give birth in hospital.' And when I was close to giving birth, that is exactly what she did, but I was just so happy at home that I stayed. I felt relaxed and comfortable. So, we called the hospital and told them what stage I was at, and if something had gone wrong, I would have been able to get to them really quickly and they'd have been prepared.

The important thing to know is that if you do want or need to go into hospital, you are NOT a failure. And if your healthcare expert is telling you to go into hospital, then you need to go to hospital because that is the safest thing for you and your baby.

I would definitely recommend finding out how long it would take to get to the hospital if you were to get transferred, because it really made a big difference to me knowing that my hospital was very close by. If you're in a town, that's obviously easier, but in the countryside, the distance might be something to take into consideration.

If you think you'd like to have a home birth, ask your midwife if this is suitable for you. Once they've given you the green light, they will make sure that all teams support you in this decision.

You can also choose to have a home birth without a midwife with you, which is called unassisted birth or free birth. Marley has explained a little more about this (see page 96). If you do have an unassisted birth, you'll need to tell a GP or your local maternity centre about your baby's birth as soon as they've been born, because by law every birth in the UK needs to be recorded within 36 hours. Your baby will also need to be seen by a doctor or midwife.

MIDWIFERY UNIT (BIRTH CENTRE)

If you are a bit worried about a home birth but would still like a more natural birth because of the reduction in possible intervention, then a brilliant choice would be a midwifery unit. Midwife-led units, also known as birth centres, or, if you're in Scotland, community maternity units (CMUs), will either be alongside a hospital maternity unit or freestanding. As the name implies, they're run by midwives, but the advantage of the centres in hospitals is that you'll have doctors and specialists very close by. However, if they're freestanding, they will be in a different place entirely, in which case they won't have any obstetric, neonatal or anaesthetic care on site.

One of the main draws of birth centres is that they feel like a less medicalised environment than a hospital. The rooms have slightly softer lighting, there is less medical paraphernalia around, and the atmosphere will feel more relaxed, like a home rather than a hospital. As with a home birth, there's also a lower chance of intervention from forceps, a ventouse or an episiotomy.

HOSPITAL BIRTH

For lots of people, a hospital feels like the safest and most comfortable option. In hospital, you'll get looked after by midwives but there is also access to other birth experts: obstetricians, anaesthetists and other specialists in newborn care if your baby needs it. They are all on hand to assist if complications arise during your labour.

Here are the things you need to take into consideration when thinking about a hospital birth:

— You might go home straight from the labour ward after recovering for a few hours, or you might be moved to a postnatal ward.

— In a hospital it's likely you'll be looked after by a different midwife from the one who looked after you during your pregnancy.

— You might be more likely to have intervention via an episiotomy, forceps or a ventouse (see pages 101, 207 and 207).

Before you make any decision, however, go and have a look at the facilities that the hospital and midwifery units offer. Ask to see a hospital room or the kind of room that you might be giving birth in. And ask loads of questions about what's available to you during labour (live performance from Chris Martin?!): do they have birthing stools/birthing pools, for example? Birthing stools are lovely. They're a little stool with a hole in it and they put your body in quite a good position to birth – a bit like squatting, but you're sitting. Sort of like sitting on the loo; really comfy. I was squatting without a stool for a long time when Holly was crowning and coming out, and it was exhausting. So, ask the midwives if it is possible to take in a birthing stool if they don't have one. Ask if you can soften the lighting or adjust the room temperature. Check if you are allowed to play music (sometimes, if it's a very busy ward and lots of women are making loud noises, it's quite nice to have music playing to distract you from that).

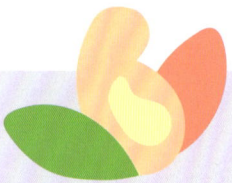

FREE BIRTH AND BBA

Midwife Marley

A free birth, also known as unassisted childbirth, is a birth that takes place without the presence or assistance of a medical professional. The birth is managed solely by the pregnant person and, in some cases, their birth partners. Free birth is a chosen path, which differs from a child born before the arrival of health professionals (BBA). A BBA may occur if a woman gives birth unexpectedly at home, in the car or elsewhere before maternity assistance can reach them. If you have a BBA and all is straightforward (i.e. there is no serious perineal trauma or excessive blood loss), you can decide whether or not to go into hospital afterwards, once you have been checked over by a midwife.

In many countries, including the UK, a woman has the legal right to choose the circumstances of her childbirth, including the option to have a free birth. This right is grounded in bodily autonomy and informed consent, meaning a woman has the authority to make decisions about her own body and medical care.

Although there is no direct evidence on the relative safety of free birth, the World Health Organization (WHO) states that skilled midwifery care during childbirth reduces the risk of neonatal and maternal morbidity and mortality. So why might someone decide to have a free birth? There are a range of reasons, including:

— **Desire for autonomy:** A wish to maintain control over the birthing process in their own safe space without being rushed or having medical intervention.

— **Negative experiences with medical births:** Previous negative experiences in hospital settings may drive women to seek an alternative.

— **Belief in natural birth:** A philosophical or spiritual belief that birth is a natural process that does not require medical intervention.

The Royal College of Midwives reported on the increase in free births during the COVID-19 pandemic, when home-birth services were cut. Some women were worried about the prospect of not being allowed to have their partners in the hospital room with them during their entire birth experience, including afterwards, and about them being told to go home. These women decided to give birth without assistance instead.

For anyone considering a free birth, my suggestion would be to discuss it with a midwife, who will be able to talk to you about your pregnancy and any things you may need to consider while making your decision. There is lots of information about free birth online – a good place to start is birthrights.org.uk, which has a fact sheet about freebirth, and the website of Dr Sara Wickham (sarawickham.com), a midwifery researcher and educator who has lots of information about making decisions during pregnancy.

Free birth is a legal right in many places and is a deeply personal choice. Many parents have reported extremely positive experiences of it. However, it is crucial to weigh up the benefits and risks carefully and to be well prepared for all potential outcomes.

A woman has the legal right to choose the circumstances of her birth, and the authority to make decisions about her own body and medical care.

YOUR STORIES

'I really struggled with having to adapt my identity.' — Helen

I felt that I was making compromises while my husband carried on with his life just as it had always been. Exercise, diet , alcohol, socialising, body image .. mine all had to change whilst he remained the same. Resentment. This is the only way I can describe it. It feels like being held in limbo due to the fact that you don't identify as your pre-pregnancy self yet you aren't a mother yet either. Getting dressed up and not feeling admired and sexy because my figure and identity in society had changed was also very hard to adapt to. Exercise is and always has been incredibly important. I visited the gym every other day but felt judged because I wasn't adopting the stereotypical 'pregnant woman' mentality. I felt that I carried all of this alone because my body and identity was the only one affected.

Davina: Helen, this is so great to read. And I don't mean that I'm happy that you struggled with your identity. I did too. Just reading your story is very comforting to anybody that struggles. I felt like my body had been taken over by an alien. It was very difficult, so thanks for your honesty. We really appreciate it.

YOUR STORIES

'I don't think I realised how powerless I'd feel.' — Sam, dad

From the outside, I looked calm – holding bags, decorating, asking questions, going to appointments. But inside, I was bracing for impact. Every appointment felt like it came with a warning. Every twinge or silence sent my mind spiralling. She was the one carrying everything – physically, emotionally. But I was carrying it too, just in a different way. The worry. The pressure to stay strong. The constant second-guessing – was I doing enough? Saying the right things? I'd feel completely useless. I wanted to take some of it off her, but I couldn't. There were moments that caught me off guard. Seeing the scan. Feeling the kick. Letting myself picture the baby's face, but every bit of hope was tangled with fear – of losing them both, of not knowing how to fix it, of what might come next. I feel like I've changed in ways I can't really understand yet.

Davina: Sam, I think it's very easy when you're carrying a baby to forget that your partner is on this journey with you and has a whole other set of worries or anxieties to deal with around how best to help and support. It's really important to hear men's perspectives. Thanks so much.

VISITING A BIRTH CENTRE AND/OR HOSPITAL

The NHS has put together a really useful checklist of questions to ask when you visit a birth centre or hospital, and I wanted to include them here so that you can just take a screenshot of this page and have it handy during your visit.

— Are tours of the maternity facilities available before the birth?

— When can I discuss my birth plan?

— Are TENS machines available for pain relief or do I need to hire one?

— What equipment is available – for example, mats, a birthing stool or bean bags?

— Are there birthing pools?

— Are partners, close relatives or friends welcome in the delivery room?

— Are they ever asked to leave the room – if so, why?

— Can I move around in labour and find my own position for the birth?

— What is the policy on induction, pain relief and routine monitoring?

— Are epidurals available?

— What are the processes for complications, when might I be transferred?

— How soon can I go home after the birth?

— What services are provided for premature or sick babies?

— Who will help me if I choose to formula feed?

— Will my baby be with me all the time or is there a separate nursery?

— Are there any special rules about visiting?

— How long would it take if I needed to be transferred to hospital from a birth centre?

— Which hospital would I be transferred to?

— Would a midwife be with me all the time?

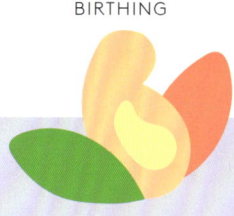

WRITING A BIRTH PLAN

Midwife Marley

Writing down your birth preferences, also called a birth plan, can be an empowering process for expectant parents, providing clarity and communication about their preferred choices for labour and birth. I like to use the term 'birth preferences', as it may leave you feeling a little deflated if your plan doesn't go as you wanted. Writing a plan is not essential, but it can help those around you to understand what you'd like, without the need to continually verbalise during labour. Noting down your preferences allows you to detail a range of scenarios in labour, and what your wishes and choices are during any particular event. Childbirth can be unpredictable, so it's good to have all bases covered.

A birth plan does not have to be extensive; just include the things that are most important to you. In many standard birth-plan templates, there may be questions that you are unsure of – for example, 'What position do you want to give birth in?' Questions like this are often impossible to answer, as you probably won't know until the time comes. For this type of question, you might opt to say something like, 'I want to be left to adopt a position that feels instinctive and comfortable for me.'

Ideally, wait until you have taken a course of antenatal classes before completing your birth preferences. You can then discuss them with your midwife at some point during your third trimester and the birth plan should then be shown to the midwife assigned to caring for you in labour. Your birth partner should be familiar with your wishes and wants, too. Start with the basic information, including your and your birth partner's names, birthplace preference, estimated due date, medical conditions and allergies.

Additional things to consider include:

LABOUR

— **Environment:** Lighting, music, and room set-up, including whether you're hoping to have a water birth. Have you practised hypnobirthing techniques? If so, let the midwives know as you are likely to appear much calmer on the outside than someone who hasn't!

— **Pain relief:** What are your thoughts on pain relief (see page 186)? Are you open to seeing what you may need, if anything, or are you set on a particular method of pain management?

— **Mobility:** Do you want to explore any birth aids if the setting has them, such as balls or birthing stools? Consider moving around in labour and how that might look if you have an epidural (see page 189). Epidurals can make the legs feel numb, making it difficult to move much. Does the hospital offer low-dose epidurals that allow some movement?

— **Vaginal and cervical checks:** Specify how you feel about vaginal and cervical checks during labour. If you're not comfortable with frequent cervical checks to monitor dilation, you could request that they be done only when essential or with your consent.

BIRTH

— **Second stage (the birth of the baby):** Do you have any preferences for this stage (i.e. waiting for spontaneous pushing, rather than being coached)?

— **Partner involvement:** Do you want your partner to be involved during the birth (i.e. 'catching the baby')? If you do, discuss this possibility with the midwife.

— **Episiotomy:** Episiotomy is a cut to the perineum, which is carried out by the midwife or obstetric doctor during the birth of the baby's head (for more information, see page 195). Write your thoughts around episiotomy. Consider that, with assisted birth (see below), this is much more likely.

— **Assisted birth:** What are your thoughts on the use of forceps (see page 207) or ventouse (see page 207)? Should it be suggested? This is commonly discussed if the pushing stage has gone on for a long time and the baby needs to be born quickly, or if the baby's head is in an awkward position.

— **Unplanned caesarean:** What are your thoughts on a caesarean (see page 211) if one is required? Who will support you in theatre?

AFTER BIRTH

— **Contact with baby:** Preference for immediate skin-to-skin contact (see page 217) or otherwise.

— **Placenta:** Do you want a managed (with an injection) or physiological (natural) third stage? If you have any plans for the placenta, such as encapsulation, mention that here so that it's not discarded. Placenta encapsulation is the process of steaming, dehydrating and grinding the placenta into a powder, which is then placed into capsules for consumption. Some believe it may offer benefits such as improved postpartum recovery, increased energy and enhanced milk production. However, scientific evidence supporting these benefits is limited.

— **Cord clamping:** Who will cut the cord and what are your thoughts on optimal cord clamping (see page 182)?

— **Sex of baby:** Do you know the sex of the baby? If not, do you want to find out yourself or for the midwife to tell you?

— **Feeding:** Your feeding preferences, i.e. whether you plan to breastfeed or formula feed (see page 248).

— **Vitamin K:** Your preference for vitamin K, which is offered to all newborns to prevent bleeding conditions. It's available via injection at birth, or orally over several doses.

— **Hospital/birth centre stay:** Are you hoping for an early discharge or are you happy to stay longer?

If you are planning a home birth, include all of the above. Do make provisions for your preferences in the event of a transfer into hospital. Your home-birth midwife will give you all the information you need regarding environment set-up and things you'll need to prepare for a home birth.

If you have any specific cultural practices/preferences surrounding childbirth, be sure to detail them here, too.

Writing a birth plan is a valuable exercise that can help ensure your experience aligns with your preferences as closely as possible. It promotes clear communication with your healthcare team and allows you to be more prepared for the birth of your child. While it's important to remain flexible, having a written plan can provide peace of mind and a sense of empowerment.

CHOOSING YOUR BIRTHING PARTNER

For many of you reading this, it might be very obvious who you want to have by your side at the birth of your baby. But for others, it might be a complicated issue.

First things first, it is almost unthinkable in today's society not to have your partner or co-parent present at the birth of your baby, but I think it's so important to acknowledge that they might not actually want to be there. For many partners, labour and birth can be an extremely traumatic time. If you're with somebody who thinks that they're going to have a bit of a meltdown or freak out about you being in pain, who doesn't want to see any blood or a placenta, and who thinks they're going to have to leave or start retching partway through, then I think they should have the option **not** to be there. Maybe they want to sit outside and be called in once the baby has arrived. Maybe they want to be with you at the beginning, for the first part of your labour, and not for the crowning or pushing out. If that's the case, try and be understanding. I know it might be disappointing. Get someone else to step in who will support you and make sure you have everything you need.

I really think this is an important thing to talk about with your partner, to show that you are willing to hear what they have to say. It's important from your perspective, too, because, if for example, your partner doesn't really want to be there, and you're in labour, in the zone, and they are not behaving in a way you need them to (i.e. they're struggling or squirming), then it's really going to get on your tits. So, do consider having an honest conversation beforehand if you sense they're worried about the birth, which might go something like this: 'Let's talk about when I give birth. What do you think you'd like to do?' They might say, 'What do you mean?' And you could say, 'What would be the perfect birth for you? Would you like to be there the whole time? Some of the time? Or would you like to wait outside and be called in when the baby arrives? I'm very happy to find somebody else who really wants to be there. And I'm not saying that you don't want to be there, just that it's in all of our interests that we ALL feel comfortable when this baby comes. And I promise you, I'm not going to freak out or feel angry with you, or take it out on you, whatever you say.' (You have to really mean that and you have to stick by it or they will never trust you again.) So, if they say, 'I really don't want to be there, I'm so worried,' you say, 'I totally understand. You can change your mind at any time, but for now I will get somebody else to be my birthing partner, for a bit of extra support.'

If you go down this route, or if you don't have a partner and need to choose a birthing partner, that person could be anybody you love or care about. They could be a friend who's had four babies and really knows what they're doing; a parent; a mother-in-law. It could be anybody you feel comfortable with and who will be present, engaged, helpful, supportive, calm and encouraging during your labour.

A birthing partner also needs to be somebody you can talk through your birth plan with, to make sure they are on board with everything that you would like to happen. What you don't want while you're in labour is a birthing partner who says to you, 'Do you think that's a good idea? Do you think we should do that?'

Your birthing partner could also be a doula. A doula is someone who supports women through their pregnancy, labour and birth, and sometimes after the baby has arrived, too. They do not have to be medically trained and can't provide medical care, but they can provide practical and emotional support. They can be your only birthing partner, or you can have them as well as your birthing partner. Often, they will answer questions you have, help you with your birth plan and then afterwards with breastfeeding or any other concerns you have as a new mum. You generally have to pay to have a doula, but there are charities out there offering free doula support for people in vulnerable situations. Doula UK provides lots more information on the options available to you, how to find a doula and who will be right for you. While doulas can be a huge help, what I would say is that it is nice to also have somebody there who you know well, to share in the moment of absolute joy just after your baby is born.

YOUR STORIES

'I thought the second trimester was meant to be the easy one. But no one told me about the insomnia.' — Dina

I'd lie in bed wide awake at 2am, feeling like my body was buzzing. Was the baby okay? Had I drunk enough water? Was I being ridiculous for googling 'what does it mean if I only feel kicks on one side?' I tried everything – warm milk, magnesium spray, even a podcast where someone talked about trains in a monotone voice (it weirdly helped). But mostly, I lay there in the dark, watching the minutes tick by. It was the weight of the unknown.

Everyone asks how you're feeling, but no one asks if you're sleeping.

Davina: Dina, isn't it funny how the second trimester is when you're kept awake? I often wondered whether that was Mother Nature trying to prepare me for how I would feel after I'd had my baby. Thanks for the tips on other ways that you can help your sleep, hygiene. Big hugs.

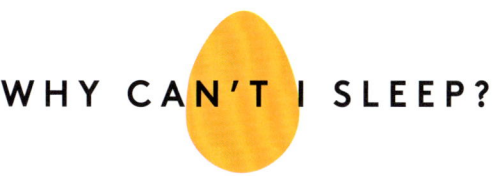

WHY CAN'T I SLEEP?

I am famous for being able to put my head on a pillow, close my eyes and be out for the count straight away (I know, it's really annoying). But not being able to get to sleep and waking up several times in the night was something I experienced during pregnancy, so I know how debilitating it is and what those nights spent overthinking feel like.

I also know that these days there's a much greater awareness of the significant role sleep plays in our overall health and wellbeing. Like exercise, it really is so important – even more so at a time when you're growing a little person inside you. Sleep is the time when our body repairs itself; it supports our immune system and controls how our body reacts to insulin, and therefore affects whether we might be more likely to develop gestational diabetes (see page 146). And yet there are several reasons why you might experience troubled sleep during your pregnancy.

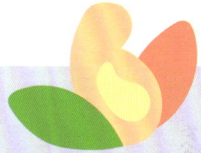

THE CAUSES OF SLEEP DISRUPTIONS

Midwife Marley

Significant sleep disruptions in pregnancy are common and can be exhausting. This is a bit of a paradox, as we know that sleep is essential in supporting the growing body and baby, yet the changes that happen to the body during pregnancy can prevent many women being able to get the restful sleep they need, which can be particularly difficult if they are going to work and/or caring for other children. So, what might be causing the restless nights?

YOUR HORMONES

During pregnancy, the body experiences fluctuations in hormone levels, including increased progesterone, which can contribute to feelings of sleepiness during the day but fragmented sleep at night. During late pregnancy, oxytocin (see page 169), the hormone responsible for contractions during labour, increases, which can also affect night-time sleep.

DISCOMFORT

Physical discomfort may prevent you from getting restful sleep. As the uterus expands to accommodate your growing baby, the pressure can cause back pain, pelvic discomfort and frequent urination. These can make it challenging to find a comfortable sleeping position and may disrupt sleep quality, particularly if you are hopping out of the bed numerous times throughout the night to go to the toilet.

RESTLESS LEG SYNDROME (RLS)

Restless leg syndrome (RLS) is another common annoyance that is often reported as being bothersome at night. It's characterised by uncomfortable sensations in the legs and an uncontrollable urge to move them. Having legs that you can't keep still can make it difficult to relax and fall asleep. No one knows exactly what causes RLS in pregnancy, but it's thought that vitamin and mineral deficiencies and hormonal fluctuations may be contributing factors. Lots of women who suffer with RLS have found relief by taking calcium or magnesium supplements. If you suffer with RLS and are thinking of trying supplements, please do discuss this with your care provider first.

HEARTBURN OR ACID REFLUX

The burning sensations that occur in the chest from heartburn/acid reflux can intensify when lying down, making it uncomfortable to sleep and causing interruptions throughout the night. Thankfully not everyone will suffer from it, but when it does occur, it isn't a nice feeling. It can occur at any time during pregnancy, but is more likely in the third trimester.

ANXIETY

It's not uncommon to experience anxiety and/or stress during pregnancy, particularly for first-time mothers or those with concerns about their health or the health of their baby. These emotional factors can contribute to insomnia, as your mind is constantly ticking over. Guided meditations may help with this, and practising breathing techniques – as Davina and Dr Louise Oliver spoke about earlier (see pages 34–37) – can also be useful. Vivid and bizarre dreams are also very common; I've heard many accounts of women having nightmares when they never usually do. This could be a result of apprehension and anxiety about the impending arrival.

WHAT POSITION SHOULD YOU SLEEP IN?

You may be wondering what the ideal way to sleep is during pregnancy, and the answer depends on what stage of pregnancy you're at, and how comfortable you're feeling. During the first trimester, you'll probably sleep no differently to how you did pre-pregnancy. As your bump starts to grow, lying on your front might feel uncomfortable, so changing your position to lie on your side is recommended.

During the late second and third trimester, lying flat on your back should be avoided where possible, as the size of the baby and uterus can put pressure on vessels supplying blood to the uterus and the rest of the body, which can result in dizziness, shortness of breath or low blood pressure, and may affect the amount of oxygen reaching the baby. Some people find that sleeping on their side is equally uncomfortable if they suffer from hip pain. If this is the case for you, try placing a pillow between your knees. If that doesn't help and sleeping on your back is the only way to get some sleep comfortably, keep slightly elevated, with a couple of pillows behind your back so that you are in a semi-sitting position.

If you go to sleep lying on your side and wake up in the night flat on your back, don't worry too much, just roll back on to your side.

Maintaining a relaxing evening routine may help you get a better night's rest. Having a warm bath, not eating big meals at night, playing meditation music and avoiding late-night screen time can all support your body and mind in winding down.

STRESS AND SLEEP

If you're not sleeping because of stress and anxiety, I totally understand. I was very anxious throughout my first pregnancy, not least because the world can be quite a stressful place, and can sometimes feel a very dangerous place. Holly was born on 22 September 2001, which was shortly after the Twin Towers had been hit in New York. And I just wept and wept and wept for the two weeks after it happened, because I thought, *What am I bringing a child into?* I think I was just super-stressed and scared, and those things aren't conducive to a calm, relaxed birth. It's almost as if, while you are pregnant, you just need to park everything, and just focus on keeping yourself well and calm, and taking care of your baby.

Concentrate on those things as much as you can – I know that's hard; we will do absolutely anything to ensure the safety and wellbeing of the little life inside of us, yet we might not go the extra mile for ourselves. So please look after yourself, and enlist other people's support to help you do that.

Mindfulness is a tool I have found so helpful at stressful times. It's all about training your mind to focus on the present moment, and I've practised it on and off for about ten years now. It really came into its own during that first COVID lockdown in 2020. Work was on hold, and I'd lie in bed at night feeling anxious about the state of the world or wake up early with a knot in my stomach. I had to do things for my sanity's sake, so I started doing mindfulness again to quiet my overactive brain and help me drift off. I downloaded the Headspace app and did guided meditations for about 10-20 minutes every day. It was amazing: I could definitely feel my mental state shifting, my worn-out batteries recharging, and I wouldn't be awake for hours in the night.

We've also provided breathing techniques (see pages 34-37) and other relaxation tips throughout the book to help you calm your mind, so please know you are not alone in managing stresses, fears and anxieties and do seek out tools to help yourself get a good night's sleep. When I was having trouble sleeping during pregnancy, I was given the technique on the next page to try (apparently, it's based on an army technique), and it really did help me, so if you're having the same experience, do give it a try.

> You are not alone in managing stresses, fears and anxieties – do seek out tools to help you get a good night's sleep.

MY ARMY-INSPIRED SLEEP TECHNIQUE

STEP 1

Lie on your side with a pillow between your legs.

Some experts believe that lying on your left-hand side enhances kidney function, which means you eliminate waste products from the body better and may experience less swelling in your feet, ankles and hands.

STEP 2

Whichever side you're on, get yourself comfortable.

Take a deep breath in through your nose and out through your nose.

STEP 3

Now you are going to send your body to sleep, starting with your toes.

Give them a little wriggle and think, *My toes are very relaxed and they're going to sleep.* Then move to the balls of your feet, and really feel them relaxing after a hard day of walking, taking all the tension out of them. Then go to your insteps and up into the arches of your feet and feel that they're relaxing. Go to your heels – your feet now feel totally heavy and relaxed. Move the thought to your ankles, which have been working all day to keep you upright, and let them fully relax, then move on to your calf muscles. Carry on, from your calves to your knees, to your quads, to your hamstrings, to your bottom. To your womb, to the baby, to the placenta. Think about all that relaxation and goodness going into the baby to keep it calm and help it go to sleep. Then move your thoughts to your chest, your lungs, breathing calmly and slowly.

STEP 4

If you're feeling tense at this point, try breathing in for four counts, and out for longer – say, six or eight counts.

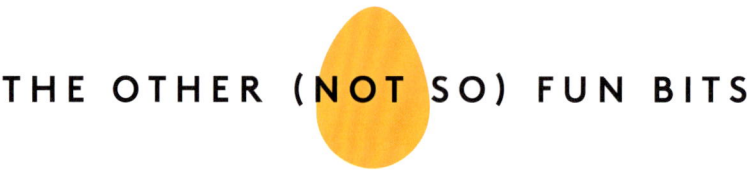

THE OTHER (NOT SO) FUN BITS

Judging from my own experience, and from those of friends and other women I speak to, it seems as though there is this widespread, somewhat misguided belief that women sail through their pregnancy once they hit the second trimester. That they develop beautiful skin, look rosy-cheeked and healthy, and positively radiate with the famous pregnancy glow (there is actually some science behind that; the hormonal changes our bodies undergo and the increased blood flow during pregnancy can cause some women to develop a particularly glowy, radiant complexion).

And yet I remember thinking, *At what point am I supposed to glow?* I just wasn't one of those people.

The reality is that for me and many women, pregnancy does not exactly make you look red-carpet ready. We've already talked about morning sickness (see page 64) and below Marley has outlined some of the other more common things that you may experience over the course of your pregnancy.

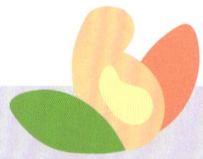

COMMON COMPLAINTS

Midwife Marley

While many women's pregnancies are plain sailing and they won't experience even a hint of nausea or heartburn, others may display every possible symptom of growing a baby. I've broken down some of the most common pregnancy complaints.

DIARRHOEA AND VOMITING

During pregnancy, vomiting and diarrhoea can be uncomfortable symptoms that can happen for a variety of reason and at different times. Aside from hyperemesis gravidarum (see page 65), pregnancy-related vomiting or diarrhoea may be brought on by hormones, changes in food tolerance and stress. (Food poisoning is also a cause of diarrhoea, so be sure to follow safe eating practices.) These signs might also come with a fever, tummy ache and feeling dehydrated.

If you're dealing with diarrhoea and vomiting while pregnant, it's really important to keep hydrated by sipping lots of fluids, especially water or drinks with electrolytes, and try nibbling on small, plain meals whenever you can. But if these symptoms stick around or get worse, or you notice other worrying signs like a fever, tummy pain or reduced baby movements, it's super-important to get medical help quickly to make sure both you and your baby are okay.

Diarrhoea that occurs close to your due date could indicate that the body is preparing for labour. This sometimes happens because the cervix releases more prostaglandins at this time, which in turn can cause contractions in your intestines. Prostaglandins are a group of fats, also known as lipids, that have hormone-like properties. They are often produced at the site of tissue damage or infection, but at the end of pregnancy, they are produced around the cervix to help it dilate.

Diarrhoea related to labour is usually short-lived, so if you experience it just keep yourself hydrated and rested. If you are feeling unwell, have severe abdominal pain or vomiting alongside the diarrhoea, call your maternity unit for advice. Stomach bugs and food poisoning can happen to anyone, even when pregnant.

HEARTBURN

Heartburn is a common pregnancy symptom that is more prevalent in the second and third trimesters. It is primarily caused by the increase in progesterone relaxing the valve between the oesophagus and stomach. This relaxation allows stomach acid to flow back into the oesophagus, causing the burning sensation known as heartburn. As your belly grows, the uterus puts pressure on the stomach, further promoting the backflow of acid. Eating large meals, lying down soon after eating and consuming certain foods like spicy or fatty dishes can exacerbate this. Managing heartburn involves adjusting your diet and avoiding trigger foods, as well as eating smaller meals.

DISCHARGE

Throughout pregnancy, it's normal to experience shifts in vaginal discharge due to hormonal changes and increased blood flow to the pelvic region. While vaginal discharge is usually a natural part of the body's cleansing process, when pregnant, you may observe alterations in its texture, colour and volume. In early pregnancy, the increase in vaginal discharge – often transparent or milky white – is linked to the thickening of the vaginal walls and the secretion of mucus for cervical protection.

As labour approaches, or as it starts, discharge may escalate in quantity and may contain traces of blood or mucus, often referred to as a 'bloody show'. This is different to the mucus plug that will be explained later (see page 168).

However, if discharge comes with itching, burning, an unpleasant odour or changes in colour, or resembles cottage cheese, it might signal a vaginal infection, such as a yeast infection or bacterial vaginosis, which needs medical attention.

Generally, practising good hygiene, opting for breathable cotton underwear and refraining from douching can help manage normal vaginal discharge during pregnancy.

Feeling more tired than normal?

FATIGUE

Feeling more tired than normal is a common symptom during pregnancy. It can manifest at different stages due to a blend of physical, hormonal and emotional factors. In the initial weeks, increased progesterone levels can lead to feelings of drowsiness and exhaustion as the body adapts to pregnancy.

As pregnancy progresses, fatigue may escalate due to heightened blood volume, hormonal shifts and the physical strain of carrying extra weight to support foetal growth. Emotional stress, anxiety and disrupted sleep patterns can further exacerbate fatigue. There are, however, things you can do to help manage it:

— Maintain a balanced diet and be sure to keep yourself well hydrated by aiming to drink at least 2.5 litres of water per day, which is around eight glasses. This can include flavoured water, but not caffeinated or fizzy drinks. Your urine should be clear and pale, not dark.

— Prioritise rest by listening to your body.

— Participate in gentle exercise or prenatal yoga for an energy boost.

— Seek support from loved ones to alleviate stress and share daily responsibilities.

HEADACHES

A large number of the women I've cared for over the years have experienced headaches at some stage of their pregnancy. Once again, they're usually caused by hormonal fluctuations, but increased blood volume and not drinking enough water are also contributing factors. Headaches can usually be managed with paracetamol (avoid ibuprofen in pregnancy unless indicated by a doctor), but if they are severe, persistent, or accompanied by other symptoms, such as sudden swelling of the face, hands and feet, visual disturbances or chest pain, you should contact your maternity care team immediately, as they may be a sign of a more serious complication.

SWOLLEN HANDS AND FEET

Mild swelling in pregnancy, also known as oedema, is a common complaint, and is generally considered normal. It tends to affect the extremities in the late second and third trimesters and is often worse in the heat, and may be more pronounced at the end of the day. There are lots of causes of the swelling, including hormonal fluctuations, an increase in blood volume and the pressure that the expanding uterus puts on lymphatic drainage and blood vessels. Drinking lots of water, avoiding prolonged standing, resting and elevating the limbs can all help reduce mild oedema.

Severe or sudden swelling, especially if accompanied by symptoms like headaches, blurred vision, chest pain or elevated blood pressure, may indicate a more serious condition like pre-eclampsia (see page 144). If this happens, you need to get checked out by your healthcare professional.

VARICOSE VEINS

Usually occurring in the legs, varicose veins are twisted, bulging veins that can have a bluish or purple hue. Some people develop them as a result of hormonal changes that relax the blood-vessel walls and the developing uterus, which puts more pressure on the veins in the lower body. Although varicose veins can be uncomfortable, they rarely present serious health concerns and are usually accepted as a typical aspect of pregnancy. Due to the body's weight gain in the late second and third trimesters, you're more prone to varicose veins at this time. To relieve symptoms and lower the chance of developing itchy skin and soreness, you may be advised to use compression stockings and take gentle exercise. It's also advisable to maintain a healthy diet and watch your salt intake.

'I cannot put into words the joy I felt getting a positive pregnancy result after years of roller-coaster emotions each month – the trying, the hope, the misery.' — Kat

Twelve weeks into my pregnancy I noticed raised bumps on the back of my neck like sandpaper. By 18 weeks my legs felt itchy and large urticaria appeared all up them. I had a wonderful midwife who got me to see an obstetrician. They couldn't explain what was happening. Meanwhile the itching intensified, and sleep was hard to come by. The only relief was to sit with my legs in freezing-cold water. I was put on steroids and creams. The urticaria spread. I was signed off sick and slept when exhausted, as the itching wouldn't allow normal sleep. I had an awful experience with a dermatologist, who said it was an infected shaving rash (my obstetrician actually made a complaint).

I was scheduled to be induced at 37 weeks, as they wanted the baby out as soon as possible. So I had two pessaries, and four hours later my little girl was born. I was in agony and had to have a doctor's arm up inside me to contract my womb. But I didn't care. My little girl lay on my chest and the love I felt overwhelmed me. I thought the itching would surely stop after the birth and, after around a month, it finally subsided, and I enjoyed my baby.

Fifteen months later and I became pregnant again. The telltale sandpaper spots appeared on my neck and the steroids and creams started once more. Then another dermatologist suggested that it could be iron-related. I was anaemic all through my first pregnancy and no number of tablets did anything. Sure enough, after blood tests it was clear that my iron levels had plummeted again. They made the decision to try an IV iron infusion. Lo and behold, the maddening itching eased.

Davina: I'm so, so sorry, Kat. This sounds unbearable and is such a sad reminder of what we sometimes have to suffer in order to be listened to and receive treatment. Thank you so much for sharing your story, which reminds us all to keep pushing to be heard and not accepting a dismissive response from a practitioner when we can feel something is wrong.

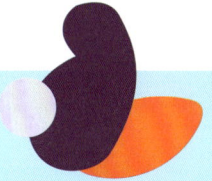

PELVIC GIRDLE PAIN
IN PREGNANCY

Jenny Gillespie, Specialist Pelvic Health Physiotherapist

Pelvic girdle pain (PGP) in pregnancy can affect around one in five women.[32] It is described as pain anywhere in the pelvis, lower back, buttocks and groin. You can start to feel pain at any point during your pregnancy, but it often starts at some time in the second trimester. Discomfort may be mild for some women; others may find it seriously affects what they are able to do, and a few may end up needing crutches or bed rest.

Common activities that you might find difficult include: standing on one leg (putting your socks on), moving your legs apart (getting into the car), turning in bed, lying on your side, climbing stairs and discomfort during sex. You would not necessarily experience all these symptoms, and your triggers may be different.[33]

The good news is that, if treated early, PGP can be managed well, reducing pain and keeping you mobile and active throughout your pregnancy.

WHAT CAUSES PGP?

Thoughts on this are changing. We used to believe that changes to your posture in pregnancy and hormonal changes potentially leading to joint laxity put more strain on the joints in the pelvis and caused pain. Now we believe that how you feel – stress, anxiety and previous experiences of pain – may play a part.[34]

Pain is not always the result of damage. Pain is processed in the same area of our brains as our emotions. If we are stressed or upset, our nervous system can be on high alert and cause our bodies to respond differently. Muscles can tighten or spasm, so we may experience higher levels of pain and there may be restrictions in movement. Education, advice and techniques to calm the nervous system response, such as breathing exercises (see the next page) and gentle movement are essential and effective ways to help manage PGP.

DEEP BREATHING/ DIAPHRAGMATIC BREATHING EXERCISES

These exercises can be a great place to start if you are experiencing some pain in pregnancy. They are also useful for helping the pelvic floor to function well.

The diaphragm (your breathing muscle, which sits underneath your lower ribs) is closely linked to your core and pelvic floor muscles and helps them work effectively. As you breathe in, your diaphragm lowers and brings about a lowering of the pelvic floor, too, helping it to relax. This is important as the pelvic floor needs to be able to move through its full range of movement to work at its best.

Breathing in this way is also very relaxing. It helps your nervous system calm its 'fight or flight' response, which occurs when you are stressed or anxious, making it really helpful for controlling pain responses and overwhelming feelings for all mums and mums-to-be.

— **Step 1** Find a comfortable position. It can be lying or sitting.

— **Step 2** Carry out a quick body scan to try to release any tension you may be holding on to.

— **Step 3** Slowly breathe in, gently expanding your lower ribs in all directions, like inflating a balloon.

— **Step 4** Pause, then gently breathe out. Your tummy should stay relaxed.

— **Step 5** Try to breathe in for a count of three and out for four or five if you can.

— **Step 6** Practise this for at least five minutes a day.

MANAGING PGP

If you are experiencing PGP, you can ask your midwife or GP to refer you to a physiotherapist, or you can find a practitioner local to you here: www. thepogp.co.uk/patients/physiotherapists

Your physio will help you to understand why you are feeling pain and give you lots of practical advice on how to manage it. They will teach you exercises that can help and may offer manual therapy and a support belt to help with the pain.[35,36]

It is important to try to manage your stress: ask for help at work or with other children if you can. Try to add some regular breath work or meditation into your day. Remain as active as you can, even if that is just some movement that feels good, or a short walk. A pillow between your knees at night can help you get comfortable, and doing pelvic-floor and core exercises can help support your pelvis.

The good news is that for most women, PGP resolves as soon as they give birth.[37] Similarly, most women with PGP manage well in labour and are able to attempt a vaginal delivery if they choose to. You may wish to consider positions for labour that may be more comfortable, like kneeling up on the bed, lying on your side, standing or going on all fours. Try to avoid lying on your back or positions where your legs are apart. You can discuss this with your midwife and add it to your birth plan (see page 91).

Pelvic girdle pain (PGP) in pregnancy can affect around one in five women.

It is described as pain anywhere in the pelvis, lower back, buttocks and groin.

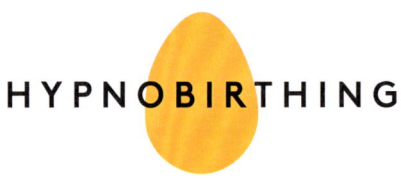

HYPNOBIRTHING

When I gave birth to my children, hypnobirthing wasn't really a thing – nobody spoke about it much – but it certainly is a thing now. It's a childbirth education method that focuses on using self-hypnosis, relaxation techniques, affirmations and breathing exercises to create a calm and positive birthing experience. What's funny is that I think I was hypnobirthing through all of my pregnancies without knowing it, but I think that if I were to go through pregnancy again, I would totally sign up to a course and learn how to do it properly. I loved all of your stories about how much hypnobirthing helped you – Jacqui, below, even describes it as her 'superpower'.

'My birthing "superpower" was given to me by a wonderful hypnobirthing practitioner.' — Jacqui

YOUR STORIES

My husband and I went to hypnobirthing sessions together during my first pregnancy. Both [home] births were the most amazing experience of my body doing what it is designed to do. I learned to feel the process my body was going through without fear of discomfort and accepted that my body and my babies knew what they were doing. I am so grateful that my body allowed me to have those births. I used a TENS machine for the contractions, which was really helpful. I am glad I took up the option of gas and air, too, which is also available during a home birth; it really took the edge off the most intense stage.

Davina: There are various hypnobirthing methods, and ways that you can learn about it online. There are classes that you can go to, or you can read about it and try to learn the techniques. Marley is a trained hypnobirthing teacher, so here she explains what it's all about.

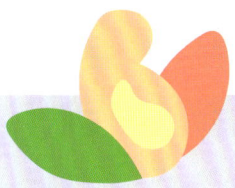

THE WONDERS OF HYPNOBIRTHING

Midwife Marley

As a hypnobirthing teacher, and someone who has used the techniques for my own births, I cannot shout loudly enough about this method! The hypnobirthing approach is designed to help you manage pain and reduce anxiety during labour and birth by promoting a state of deep relaxation and focus. Hypnobirthing has increased in popularity over the past couple of decades, and although it concentrates on promoting and nurturing the natural physiology of birth, it has been used by parents to remain calm and relaxed in all birthing scenarios, including caesareans.

One of the principles of hypnobirthing is eliminating fear and promoting confidence. Fear during labour activates our primal 'fight or flight' response (see page 116), causing stress hormones to make the heart speed up, which forces blood to the arms and legs and ultimately depletes blood flow to the uterus, creating increased uterine pain and potentially hindering the labour process. Extreme fear causes the body to become tense, and that tension prohibits the body from functioning as it should. The result is often exactly what expectant parents fear the most – long, painful birthing or unnecessary intervention.

The benefits of hypnobirthing are not just theoretical; many studies have been carried out, revealing tangible benefits including:

— reduced perception of pain

— reduced length of labour

— reduced need for medical intervention

— increased chance of a faster recovery (from any type of birth)

— calmer babies at birth

— fewer cases of post-natal depression

Hypnobirthing can be helpful for those who have had previous traumatic birth experiences, or for first-time mums who have a fear of childbirth.

Aside from teaching in depth about the physiology of birth and what's required to nurture this process, hypnobirthing employs several techniques, which you practise at home during your pregnancy, so that you're ready to use them for the birth. These include:

— **Breathing exercises:** Specific breathing techniques to help manage contractions and maintain calmness.

— **Visualisations:** Visualising positive imagery can reduce fear and anxiety.

— **Affirmations:** Positive mantras and statements reinforce confidence and empowerment.

— **Guided meditations:** Scripts read by a birth partner or played from a recording help induce a state of deep relaxation and focused concentration to manage pain and discomfort. All hypnobirthing course scripts are different, but you listen to them at home, or a partner reads them to you so that by the time you give birth, you are so used to hearing them that they should help you feel more relaxed. I offer scripts in my online hypnobirthing course but other instructors may also provide them.

— **Massage and anchors:** Birth partners will learn how to use key words or touch specific parts of the body to help keep you focused. They will learn massage techniques to help promote oxytocin release (see page 169), which is needed to help with optimal uterine contractions.

It's generally recommended to start practising hypnobirthing techniques in the second trimester, ideally around 24 weeks. This allows time for you to become comfortable with the techniques and to integrate them into your weekly routine. The techniques can be learned at any stage in pregnancy, however – it's never too late to learn.

Hypnobirthing classes come in all shapes and sizes. They may be local, face-to-face group classes, online classes or one-to-one private sessions. They may be intensive – over a day or two – or run for a couple of hours a week over several weeks. If you decide to try hypnobirthing, you'll have to decide what type of class will best fit your schedule. A teacher that provides you with a book or manual, along with affirmations and recordings for you to practise at home, is always a good option. Don't be afraid to ask any instructor questions about their course or their knowledge and experience before you sign up.

One essential component of hypnobirthing is the knowledge of birth biomechanics. Learning about the movement and alignment of the baby in relation to your body and pelvis during labour is an integral part of any childbirth/antenatal class, and practical demonstrations of exercises and positions for you to do at home should be given.

Similarly, at some point during any type of antenatal class, the teacher should explain that whatever interventions they are talking about are optional. For example, when talking about screening tests, induction of labour or vaginal examinations, the teacher should emphasise that these are all things that are offered, not just 'done'. Hypnobirthing courses don't only go into detail about practical ways to work with your body for birth; there should also be a lot of discussion about informed choice and consent. This helps with your confidence when making decisions about your care.

Being able to follow up with your instructor after a course if you have any questions is beneficial, too.

Hypnobirthing is a popular choice of childbirth education for thousands of expectant parents each year, but it is not a magic wand. It cannot guarantee a perfect experience, nor should it be assumed that hypnobirthing means zero pain. Although many women will recall their experience of hypnobirthing being far more comfortable than births they had without hypnobirthing, everyone is different. There are lots of factors that contribute to a positive birth experience and hypnobirthing should be considered part of a tool kit.

Hypnobirthing is not yet a regulated practice so a certain level of due diligence is needed when searching for a practitioner. Check for qualifications such as hypnobirthing diplomas, registered midwifery, and/or hypnotherapy.

One of the principles of hypnobirthing is eliminating fear and promoting confidence.

'It wasn't until I trained as a birth doula that I found out how important the role of oxytocin is in childbirth.' — Amie

I don't explicitly remember it being explained to me in my NCT [National Childbirth Trust] group for my first child – it may have been mentioned but I didn't take it in fully. I now understand the importance of creating a calm and safe atmosphere for this 'love hormone' to work at its best. It was explained to me in such a way that made sense: that what got the baby in there was what would get the baby out. This shy hormone needs to be given privacy, warmth, darkness – no questions or list-making or interruptions – to emerge fully. Sex needs to be given the same conditions; the two environments look and feel very similar (mostly, although some people like to be in a brightly lit hospital with medical professionals to feel safe). This information blew my mind – so much so that I wanted to go back and have more babies just to try it out. I had already had my brood by then, so had to be content with helping other families on their birth journeys.

One method of birth preparation that I felt went hand in glove with giving oxytocin its best chance of emerging was hypnobirthing. This method of feeding the subconscious with positive affirmations around birth helps to eradicate unconscious fears and has a powerful effect on the mind–body connection. I could talk for hours about birth physiology, as once this is understood, not only is the experience of giving birth changed for the better, but those who are in a supporting role can feel empowered to know how best to do this, by being guardians of the birthing space and helping to maintain a calm and safe environment for an optimal birthing experience.

Davina: Amie's words are so unbelievably powerful. I totally and utterly agree with positive affirmations during labour – they helped me so much throughout my births, and also how important the environment you give birth in is, even when you're in hospital. You can absolutely make your room a calm and peaceful space. You are the guardians of that birthing space.

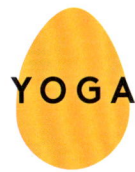

YOGA

I first met Tessa Clemson when we worked together on a documentary called *Davina McCall's Pill Revolution* about women's experience of contraception, and I spent some time in her beautiful Lancashire studio practising yoga with her and the group of women we interviewed. Although

I didn't take up yoga until after my pregnancies, I've practised yoga for years now and really feel its effects in both my body and mind. I knew Tessa was the perfect person to explain how yoga can be beneficial during pregnancy and postpartum.

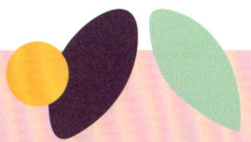

PREGNANCY YOGA

Tessa Clemson, Yoga Teacher

There are many benefits to practising yoga at any time, but it is particularly valuable in helping to prepare women for the transformative experience of meeting their baby. Pregnancy yoga is accessible whether you are a beginner or already a dedicated yogi, and the connection you build with your baby and the habits you form during pregnancy can have a lasting positive impact on your life beyond the birth.

As you progress through each stage of your pregnancy and approach your estimated delivery date (EDD), you will notice changes in your body and differences in how you feel. Pregnancy yoga helps you move instinctively throughout these stages, giving you an opportunity to slow down, reflect and tap in to your intuition as to how you feel physically, mentally and emotionally. You can start practising movements and stretches after your first scan at around 12 weeks, but the techniques of being present, focusing on your breath and connecting with your baby can be used from conception.

As your baby grows, your body adapts and your centre of gravity changes, affecting your posture and balance. Flowing through positions and practising breathing during this time builds confidence and helps you reclaim ownership of a body that can start to feel alien. This increased confidence and awareness also encourages self-advocacy and clearer communication, which are important skills to have during pregnancy.

Another benefit is that dynamic movements and positions can reduce aortic pressure (the blood pressure in the aorta component of the heart), making contractions more efficient and also increasing the opening of the pelvis.[38] Yoga positions practised during class, such as malasana (a low squat), are also active birth positions that can be used right up to and during birth, to promote optimal foetal positioning (when the baby's head is down) and create space for the baby to move through the birth canal.

Breathing techniques and visualisations taught during a pregnancy yoga class can be used in birth preparation and to work through contractions, helping to reduce anxiety, stress and tension. In times of change and uncertainty, knowing how to harness your breath can feel empowering and uplifting. Your baby can also hear your breath and the rhythm of your heart beating – and when you are relaxed, so are they.

Birth is a physiological process, and pregnancy yoga is a holistic practice that can support women in having a 'normal birth' (i.e. a natural birth that takes place without help from doctors). However, the techniques used, including the non-physical elements of yoga such as breathing and the ability to calm your mind, can be applied to all births, including assisted births and caesareans. Pregnancy yoga also aids postnatal recovery after caesarean by gently strengthening the core muscles and improving overall flexibility. The mindful breathing and relaxation techniques can reduce stress and enhance emotional wellbeing during recovery.

Up to 150 minutes of weekly exercise is recommended for pregnant women,[39] and like all exercise, yoga releases endorphins (happy, feel-good hormones), improves sleep and, if practised in a group setting, can be a great way of meeting new friends and building a support network.

Whether through physical movements, breathing techniques or visualisations, oxytocin is released when practising yoga. This powerful hormone is promoted when women feel safe, cared for and connected, and it is needed to stimulate contractions, which cause dilation of the cervix. Oxytocin also encourages the flow of breastmilk and is essential for bonding between mum and baby, especially during feeding.

Pregnancy yoga provides dedicated, uninterrupted time to bond with your baby. Babies can hear your voice and feel your touch, and research shows they can even recognise smells from their time in the womb. The things you do when practising yoga are shared experiences and can be repeated during birth and postnatally to help you feel calm, confident and comfortable. Remember, you and your baby are on this journey together, and being mindful of this can strengthen your connection with your body, your breath and your beautiful baby.

Yoga in pregnancy can also help with symptoms such as pelvic girdle pain, gestational diabetes (see page 146) and high blood pressure (hypertension). If you have any questions or concerns about any of these, it is important to seek advice from a healthcare practitioner and to attend sessions with a teacher who is fully trained in prenatal yoga.

Breathing techniques taught during a pregnancy yoga class can be used in birth preparation and to work through contractions.

FINDING OUT THE SEX OF YOUR BABY

This is an interesting one for me because I've done it both ways. On the one hand, not knowing the sex of your baby is one of life's great – and beautiful – mysteries. And I've got to say that one of the things that kept me going through pregnancy – and I wasn't a natural at being pregnant; I felt like my entire body and brain had been taken over by an alien – was the promise of a surprise, so waiting to find out the sex of my baby gave me something to hold out for. I didn't find out with Holly, but when I had Tilly, we decided we wanted to know, so at our 20-week scan, which is when you can ask to find out the sex, we were told we were having a little girl. And, actually, I have to say that it was really sweet knowing. We named her; we decorated her room; I got her lots of clothes; I was fully prepared. And, of course, I was elated when she came out, but there wasn't that 'it's a girl/it's a boy' moment, which is so exciting. It was a different feeling.

So, when I got pregnant with my third baby, I realised I'd sort of missed that 'it's a boy/it's a girl' reveal and I didn't find out. And yet it's funny, because when Chester popped out, I was so happy. I was just looking into his eyes going, 'Oh my God, it's a baby. And it's alive, and I've just given birth to it. And I'm in a pool.' I felt absolutely amazing. And then someone said to me, 'What is it?' And I wanted to go, 'It's a baby.'

And then I was like, 'Oh, I don't know what sex it is!' And I moved the umbilical cord and saw that Chester was a little boy and I just burst into tears. I just couldn't believe it. I was just so happy to have a baby. I didn't mind at all what it was, it was just so miraculous to have him.

So, basically, I'm going to sit on the fence on this one. There are reasons to find out the sex of your baby, and there are reasons not to find out. There are ways that you can find out and your partner doesn't. I know people who were given the sex of their baby in an envelope, and they didn't tell the other person involved, but you might feel weird about one of you knowing and one of you not knowing. I've had other friends who found out the sex of their baby and then told no one. Hard to keep that kind of secret, though, right? Or you can have a good old guess, so the suspense of it keeps you going. The bottom line is, you do whatever feels right for you.

RECEIVING A DIAGNOSIS OR DISCOVERING CONCERNS RELATED TO MATERNAL OR BABY'S HEALTH

Dr Caroline Boyd, Perinatal Clinical Psychologist and Author

While the myth of 'Supermum' has us believe that pregnancy is simply a happy, joyful time, the demands and changes can bring high levels of stress, anxiety and low mood, as well as physical health challenges for many mums-to-be. Receiving a maternal health diagnosis can feel overwhelming. Conditions such as high blood pressure (hypertension), pre-eclampsia, gestational diabetes, and hyperemesis gravidarum (see page 65) each bring unique challenges. These may be discovered at different points given that hospital policies may influence the timing or type of testing carried out. For example, some hospitals routinely screen for gestational diabetes while others may not.

Meanwhile an unclear diagnosis can raise anxiety. For example, concerns from maternity staff about the baby's size or foetal movement emerging later in pregnancy may lead to extra monitoring. These concerns can feel distressing, even if no evidence of increased risk is confirmed, and impact decision-making around birth.

Try to focus on what you can control. Ask your maternity team for clear, detailed information about your diagnosis or concerns and any interventions. Understanding your condition and evidence-based outcomes can help reduce uncertainty and empower you to make informed decisions about your care. Don't hesitate to ask for clarification, seek a second opinion and explore additional research if concerns are raised that don't align with your understanding.

Aspects of your pregnancy journey, with all the advice about what to eat/ what to avoid, and medicalised procedures can leave you feeling prodded, poked and 'done to', can raise anxiety and make you feel even less in control of your body. Especially when your pregnant body is already functioning differently and feeling less familiar, alongside potentially feeling physically unwell. Practise grounding techniques or gentle movement to help you find internal safety. Share how you're feeling with an empathic loved one to help you process and make sense of your emotions. For additional support, you may wish to access a perinatal therapist, via your GP, maternity team or privately, for one-to-one therapy. Seek out support groups, on and offline, that connect you with others facing similar challenges.

Receiving a prenatal diagnosis of a foetal anomaly is commonly experienced as shocking and emotionally challenging for parents. After diagnosis, parents begin a complex process as they navigate intense feelings, including shock, disbelief, fear, anger, grief, guilt and denial. These emotions are a normal, understandable response to the turn of events when plans and expectations for the birth of a longed-for healthy baby may feel broken, and the hoped-for path to parenthood takes a new direction. The task for birthing people and their partners is to process and reassess their current plans and view of the future.

Unexpected findings leading to concerns about the baby's health may give rise to complex decision-making. There may be a limited timeframe to understand the implications of the detected condition(s) to inform choices and make decisions about their baby's care. Depending on the severity and ambiguity of the diagnosis, expectant parents are more likely to experience depression, anxiety and traumatic stress. While the diagnosis itself is often experienced as traumatic, parents may be confronted with a deeply painful choice: to continue or end the pregnancy. Diagnosis of a foetal anomaly that is fatal or potentially life-threatening can trigger an intense grief reaction in parents, exacerbated by poor care and support.

This is why families need careful, non-judgmental support on a journey that brings many powerful emotions – perhaps oscillating between hope and detachment – as they adjust to their new reality. What's crucial to understand is that distress is not a sign of weakness, and experiencing conflicting emotions doesn't mean you don't love your baby or that you're a bad parent.

A diagnosis often activates a referral to a specialist clinic. Accessing information and honest, open communication from the team is essential for increasing parents' understanding and reducing uncertainty where possible. In order to feel guided and supported through difficult decision-making, what becomes essential for parents is finding a safe space to process and make sense of the news and its implications. A partner may be able to offer that space, along with other 'safe people' such as close friends or family. However, for some couples, whose cultural, religious or moral beliefs differ, it may be helpful to access a perinatal therapist to support both partners through the process of complex decision-making. For a woman who has previously experienced trauma and baby loss, or loss more generally, accessing individual therapy, if possible, via her GP or an independent therapist, may also be beneficial. Whether it's through community, peer or therapeutic support, what parents need is to make meaning of the diagnosis, and to build a sense of their baby's identity and their own parental identity, in these changing circumstances.

Deciding how and when to tell others about your diagnosis, or your baby's, is deeply personal. You may choose to share only with those closest to you or seek a wider support network. When sharing difficult news, you may find it helpful to:

— Write down what you want to say beforehand.

— Ask a 'safe person' to be present when you share the news.

— Set boundaries about what you're comfortable discussing.

> **Families need careful, non-judgmental support on a journey that brings many powerful emotions – perhaps oscillating between hope and detachment – as they adjust to their new reality.**

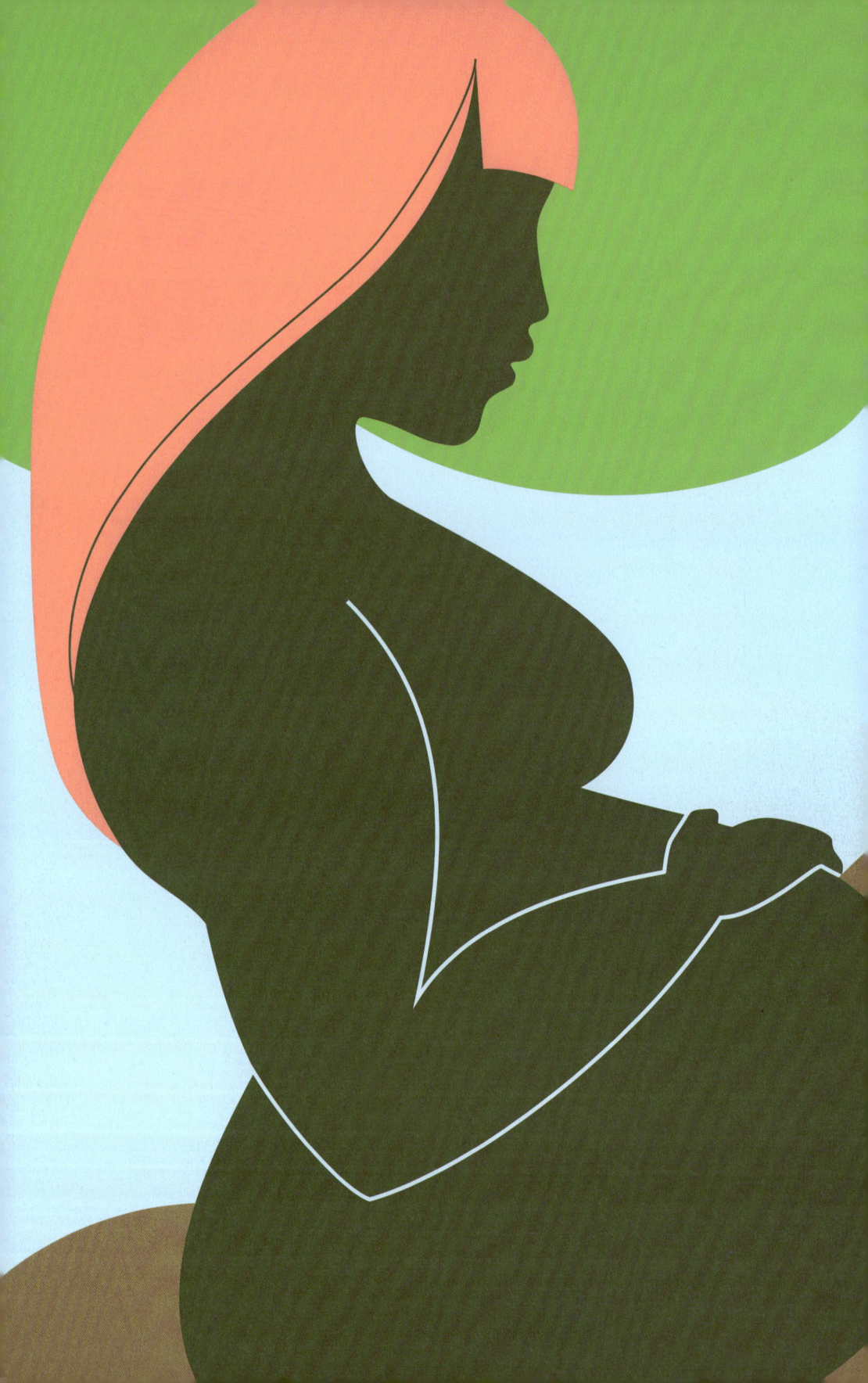

CHAPTER 4

THIRD TRIMESTER

28–40 WEEKS

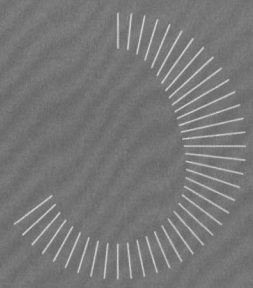

The home stretch...

PREPPING, PACKING, NESTING (AND WAITING)

This stage takes you from the 28-week mark right up until your baby is born, which in a full pregnancy is 40 weeks. At 38 weeks, your baby is considered 'full term', so theoretically they may arrive at any point. That does feel like an odd moment. I found I became hyper-aware of my body and any signs that the baby might be on its way. Everyone is going to feel differently as they approach their due date – you might feel nervous, excited, anxious or a mixture of all three, but one thing that does characterise this trimester, which is common to everyone,

is the overwhelming need to prepare as best you can. You might be starting antenatal classes, getting a nursery ready and buying the things you're going to need for your baby (see page 139), as well as packing your hospital bag (see page 141). And you might be helping to get your body primed for birth by doing perineal massage (see page 153) or harvesting your colostrum (see page 151) to help give your baby additional nourishment. And if that nesting feeling kicks in (see page 136) and you're running about the house spring cleaning like a woman possessed, as I was, you're know you're really ready to meet your baby.

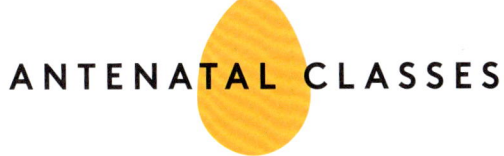

ANTENATAL CLASSES

Antenatal classes help you prepare for your baby's birth and make informed decisions about the options that might be presented to you during labour. Classes are available free on the NHS, or you can pay for them yourself, and there are lots of different options: NCT, Baby & Bump, NowBaby and Happy Parents Happy Baby are just a few.

When choosing, just think about what you are hoping to learn or gain from the classes, and look at different options so that you can find the class that will suit you, as there are differences in style and the topics covered. Most classes start when you're about 30 or 32 weeks pregnant, so about eight to ten weeks before your due date, but they can get booked up, so it's worth thinking about

booking yourself in ahead of time. Most are now available online as well as in person, but I really feel like in person is better where it's feasible. I mean, I think everything in person is better – that connection is so important.

I didn't do antenatal classes, for the same reasons I didn't give birth in a public hospital at that time – I was just too anxious about paparazzi and wanting to keep my life private and my baby out of the press, but I wonder whether I missed out. So many friends of mine are still friends with the people they met at their classes. Your kids are all born around the same time, and if you are in contracted employment, you'll have around six months to a year off and you'll probably be able to hang out together for part or all of that time – and your babies will have instant playmates.

Antenatal classes offer a source of support and camaraderie that I didn't have, and I regret that. However, as with many things, there are two sides to the coin and antenatal classes aren't for everyone. There are many women and couples who simply don't find them supportive for the type of birth they want to pursue, or feel they didn't prepare them adequately to make informed choices at the time of their birth. This is why it's so important to research the kind of classes available to you and to establish what it is you want to achieve by attending them.

I did do other things where I met other mums, though – especially postnatal classes, so things like baby massage and baby yoga. I went along to these classes and talked about my labour with others, but I'm not sure it was the same as an antenatal class because we didn't have the bonds you form through that shared experience. You've been with the people in your class for weeks, so you've already spent lots of time together, which means that after your births it's so natural and reassuring to meet up and talk about how hard you're finding everything, or just to support each other through that next stage, because everybody needs a bit of support after their baby is born. The other thing about doing antenatal classes is that partners get to meet each other, which is really great.

YOUR STORIES

'We couldn't afford the NCT classes – they were just too expensive.' — Charlotte

I remember sitting at the laptop late one night, hovering over the 'book now' button, trying to justify it to myself but my maternity cover was really low, and we were struggling to buy everything we needed so in the end we didn't go for it. Instead, we watched YouTube videos from midwives and doulas, bookmarked NHS pages, read forums full of parents swapping tips and truths. I downloaded every free app going. Some were actually brilliant – funny, reassuring, no fluff. We even did a free antenatal course at the local hospital, and the midwife running it was a gem. Straight-talking. Warm. Exactly what we needed. But I still felt the gap sometimes. Like there was this club we weren't part of. I worried we'd show up to the delivery suite underprepared. But in the end, what got us through wasn't the perfect plan – it was staying calm, listening, and trusting each other and everything was fine.

Davina: Charlotte, I'm so glad you were able to find the resources you needed and they helped support you in the right way – thank you for sharing your advice.

'I had a traumatic birth, and if I hadn't joined an NCT class, neither me nor my husband would have been prepared for what happened.' — Julie

Labour was long and problematic. I haemorrhaged and was losing a lot of blood. My daughter was born and handed straight to my husband as I was rushed to theatre. It's terrifying, but our NCT teacher had talked us through (with LEGO figures) what happens in theatre, how many people would be there, the noise, who's who. Without that information I don't think we would have coped as well as we did, *particularly my husband. We made good friends through NCT and not one of us had a straightforward birth. The support during and after was amazing.*

Davina: Julie, thanks for your story. Something that I hear time and again is that one of the greatest gifts NCT offered them was friends to hang out with, swap experiences and share the load with after their birth.

'We attended NCT classes, opting for the crash course.' — Karen

I am a nurse and my husband is a hospital consultant, but we didn't tell anyone that. The whole emphasis was on natural birth, and that if you have a caesarean or epidural, you've medicalised your birth, therefore making it unnatural in some way. There's also a massive emphasis on breastfeeding and if you didn't then you had failed.

Davina: Karen, the idea that anybody is made to feel less-than for the type of birth that they had makes me feel super sad. I think that this is a really valuable angle to hear about, and hopefully anybody who's connected to NCT will take that on board and use it to make other women's experiences better going forwards. Thank you, Karen.

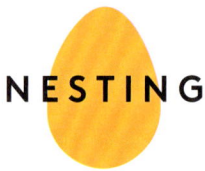

NESTING

I didn't really think nesting was a thing before I had a baby. I just thought it was a time in the lead-up to giving birth where you buy stuff for the baby, like clothes and the cot. I cannot tell you how wrong I was. For a couple of weeks before I had the baby, I felt this bizarre urge to get my life in order. I wanted to spring clean, get organised and make sure that everything had a place.

Nesting feels like an absolutely undeniable need to get your home and life ready for your new baby. I think, instinctively, your body just knows that after you've had the baby, you're not going to want to do anything except look at, love and cherish it, so you're not going to have time to do all the cleaning and the sorting – or anything else!

For me, the absolute peak of it came a couple of days before I went into labour and what was interesting was that when I was doing the cleaning and the sorting, I also put on quite loud house music and started dancing. As my midwife pointed out to me, what I was actually doing was instinctively trying to get my baby's head in the right position to give birth. It is the most incredible, intuitive thing, and it's funny because it's the same with animals: they also prepare a place that is perfect for their babies and keeps them safe from predators. It's what we do, and it is a very, very real thing.

So, if you have a partner who is nesting, go easy on her and let her do it, but more importantly help her do it, because it means that you will be providing a safe place for her and your baby. So, nesting is really a very lovely and clever biological sign that you are near the end of your pregnancy and very close to meeting your baby.

WHAT TO BUY FOR YOUR BABY – THE ESSENTIALS

What you buy for your baby and when will, of course, be very individual and depend on your budget, as well as many other factors – including when you feel ready to acknowledge that your pregnancy is progressing smoothly, as it's common for some women to feel superstitious or anxious about it right up until the final few weeks. You can start buying things at any time – and looking out for sales on baby items can be really helpful in keeping costs down – but by the third trimester, when your bump is likely to be quite prominent and nesting has potentially kicked in, you'll likely be ready to start focusing on what you need, to make sure everything is ready for your baby's arrival.

Trying to prepare for your baby can be an expensive time, and there is so much to think about, but there are things your baby will need, things you will need, and things you definitely don't, and there are a lot of things that people might make you think you need.

A baby bath is a classic one – you can very easily bath your baby in a wide sink or over your actual bath; you don't need a baby bath, so this is not an essential. For the first few weeks your baby is not going to be getting dirty, so you just give them a wash down in some nice water. You don't need to start thinking about soaps or washing hair or anything like that yet.

Something I couldn't live without, on the other hand, was giant muslins – these are amazing because they moonlight as so many different things. A giant muslin can fold up and be a blanket. In a pushchair, it can unfold and become a barrier to the sunlight that you can hang over a pram if your baby's sleeping. It can be something you might lay on the ground for your baby to lie on. It's something you put over your shoulder if your baby is sick. It's something you can swaddle the baby in. So there are many, many things you can do with them and that's kind of what you want – pieces of equipment that can multitask. So I can't recommend those highly enough.

Another thing that I found invaluable – though it's not an 'essential' as such – is a sling or carrier to carry your baby against your chest. I literally spent my first three months carrying each baby on me. Sometimes you'll want to do housework and walk around the house and a baby just loves feeling safe and warm near you, so I used mine constantly, but you might feel differently.

My children all loved their black-and-white books, and research suggests there are developmental reasons for this.[29] When babies are born, their retina is not yet fully developed, and they can only see around 25 to 30cm in front of them. Showing them contrasting shapes and patterns is thought to help stimulate their visual development, and as black and white is the starkest contrast, they register most strongly on a baby's retina, enabling them to see shapes and defined forms in a world that is otherwise quite blurry. Stronger visual signals mean more brain growth and faster visual development.

Instead of buying everything new, consider buying certain things second-hand. Charity shops and eBay often have very good things, and given that newborns grow out of everything really quickly, they will be almost brand new. The NCT do nearly-new sales of second-hand toys, essentials and baby clothes, and there are loads of really good sites online. These are just a few that I recommend checking out:

— **The Octopus Club** (theoctopusclub.com) is a pre-loved marketplace for all things baby, children, maternity – they have clothing, as well as sleeping and other equipment, such as buggies.

— **Second Snuggle** (secondsnuggle. co.uk) sells pre-loved clothing, maternity wear and toys.

— **Rascal Babies** (rascalbabies.co.uk) restores and sells used pushchairs, prams and other baby equipment, including car seats, toys, nursery equipment and lots more.

Wherever and however you choose to shop, I've put together a list opposite of the items I felt were essential to have in preparation for the first few months of your baby's life, as well as the things that were just 'nice to have' – those things that help ease things a little for you, or are sweet additions to your baby's world, but you can absolutely manage without them. They're quite often things that make nice gifts so if anybody is wondering what to get you, they might make useful suggestions.

Life is incredible for a newborn – there's so much to look at! – so there isn't a huge need for toys and teddy bears, but obviously people might want to buy you these things, which is lovely.

Trying to prepare for your baby can be an expensive time, but there are things you and your baby will need, and things you definitely don't.

Bedding

ESSENTIALS

Moses basket or crib

3–4 fitted sheets

Waterproof cover

Blanket

Baby's sleeping bag (buy the correct tog for the time of year of your birth; they come in two weights – winter or summer)

Clothing

ESSENTIALS

10–15 short-sleeved bodysuits

10–15 long-sleeved babygrows/sleepsuits

2–4 pairs of scratch mittens

3–4 hats

3–5 pairs or socks

3–5 wool/cotton cardigans depending on the season

Cleaning

ESSENTIALS

Nappies

Unscented disposable wipes

Barrier/nappy rash cream

Soft cotton towels

NICE-TO-HAVES

Changing mat

Baby bath

Feeding

ESSENTIALS	NICE-TO-HAVES
Breast pump (I highly recommend the manual ones but you can get electric)	I needed breast pads because every time I thought about my baby and the baby wasn't with me, or heard someone else's baby cry, I would start leaking, it was insane!
Breastmilk storage bags	
Bottles and sterilising equipment	Nipple cream (my nipples weren't too bad but some people's nipples really crack)
Formula (if you know you're going to be formula-feeding)	
Muslin cloths	
Bibs	

Travel

ESSENTIALS	NICE-TO-HAVES
Car seat	Baby sling or wrap
Travel bag	Baby carrier
Pram	

Other

ESSENTIALS	NICE-TO-HAVES
Sanitary pads for you	Baby rocker
Nursing bras	

WHAT TO PACK IN YOUR HOSPITAL/BIRTH CENTRE BAG

It's a good idea to have your hospital bag packed a few weeks before your due date just in case your baby comes early. Let your birth partner or whoever is driving you to the hospital or birth centre know where the bag is and what's in it, and just have it sitting in your bedroom or where nobody's going to move it. You'll need things for you and for your baby. Your birth partner might be in the hospital or birth centre for a long time – possibly even overnight – so it's helpful to have some things packed for them, too.

I've put together a list below of some of the key items you might want to pack. Some of them might seem quite obvious, but believe me it's really useful to have thought about them now and be ready to go, as you won't be able to focus on getting anything together once your contractions have started. These are the things that I put in mine (in case I had to go into hospital), but what you need might look different. Have a chat to friends and other mothers about what they took with them.

FOR YOU

- [ ] Your birth plan

- [ ] A comfy, loose outfit for labour (if you're not already wearing it when you leave; a spare is a good idea)

- [ ] A dressing gown, some comfy slippers, maybe some kind of loose tracksuit

- [ ] Your wash bag with all your essential toiletries, including any medications you're taking

- [ ] Dry shampoo is really useful if you don't want to wash your hair

- [ ] Hair ties

- [ ] Your glasses or contacts

- [ ] A phone charger and cord (the longest cord you have, because the plugs are often miles away, or an extension cable)

- [ ] Two or three bras, including a nursing bra or tank top (if you're planning to breastfeed)

- [ ] Breast pads

- [ ] A set of pyjamas suitable for breastfeeding (comfy and with easy access for your baby to feed)

- [ ] Five or six pairs of knickers

- [ ] A pack of maternity pads or five or six pairs of postpartum knickers (I didn't realise how much you bleed after giving birth, and these are ideal for absorbing the blood without the itchiness that maternity pads sometimes have)

- [ ] A loose-fitting, really comfy going-home outfit that you keep clean until you leave the hospital/birth centre

- [ ] A pillow

- [ ] A blanket or something to keep you warm (sometimes hospital rooms can be weirdly cold)

- [ ] A towel (hospitals only supply baby towels)

- [ ] A TENS machine if you're using one

- [ ] A bikini for the pool (if you don't want to be naked)

- [ ] Flip-flops (if you need to use the hospital shower and are funny about things like that – I am)

- [ ] Healthy snacks

- [ ] Water bottle

- [ ] Straws if you are planning a caesarean or in the event of an emergency, as it's easier to drink through them

- [ ] Earplugs and/or an eye mask (if, like me, you find it hard to sleep around noise)

- [ ] Books/magazines/podcasts (stuff to help you pass the time and distract you if you need that)

- [ ] Your birth playlist (this is a fun one – you and your partner deciding what you want to give birth to; I've heard of people giving birth to some very funny tracks)

FOR YOUR BABY

- [ ] Two or three sleepsuits

- [ ] Two or three outfits (bodysuits and vests; if you do have to stay in hospital for more than a night, your partner, your parents or a friend will be able to go home and get you some more, but you'll need a few with you because babies will often poo or wee when you're changing their nappy at the beginning)

- [ ] Muslins (as I've said, I love the extra-large ones)

- [ ] Hat (even in summer, babies need to feel protected and sometimes in the hospital they might want a little hat on)

- [ ] A blanket

- [ ] Water-based wet wipes (try to find the biodegradable ones) or cotton-wool balls (which you then moisten)

- [ ] Nappies (whichever type you're choosing to use)

- [ ] A warm outfit for the baby to go home in (a bodysuit and vest, plus an extra layer if you're giving birth in the winter)

- [ ] If you're planning on formula-feeding from the start, bring milk and sterilised bottles, as the hospital won't provide these. They will only provide milk to breastfeeding mothers in situations where they are struggling to feed their baby.

- [ ] Harvested colostrum (see page 151) if you've done that (it has to be named and dated for the hospital fridge)

- [ ] Car seat, even if you'll be travelling by taxi or getting a lift from a friend/family

FOR YOUR BIRTH PARTNER

- [ ] Cash for the car park (not all hospitals or centres will take cards for parking yet)

- [ ] Change of clothes and some wash things

- [ ] Snacks for them so they don't have to keep leaving you if they are hungry

- [ ] I know this is a short list so here's an extra one: help your partner!

COMPLICATIONS IN PREGNANCY

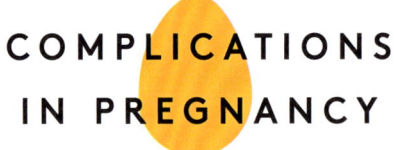

Sometimes things can go wrong in pregnancy, and you and your baby need to be given extra care and monitoring, particularly during the latter stage of your term. There's often no rhyme or reason for a complication arising, but you will be at greater risk if you have some kind of pre-existing medical condition, such as diabetes, cancer, anaemia or epilepsy. Early detection and prompt treatment will help manage complications, so if you have any doubts or concerns about how you're feeling, please make sure you discuss them with your healthcare provider, however insignificant a symptom might feel to you. The number of medical appointments ramps up during the third trimester, so you should have more opportunities to raise any worries. Marley has outlined here the symptoms and signs of the most common types of complication that can occur, but there are many others, which is another reason why it's good to flag anything unusual.

PRE-ECLAMPSIA

Marley: Pre-eclampsia is a serious and potentially life-threatening condition that can occur during pregnancy, characterised by high blood pressure and potential damage to organs such as the kidneys and liver. In the UK, pre-eclampsia affects approximately 2 to 8 per cent of pregnancies, making it one of the most common complications. Pre-eclampsia most commonly occurs during the third trimester, but can occasionally develop before this, as early as 20 weeks in extremely rare cases. One of the ways we can detect signs of pre-eclampsia is through testing your urine and blood pressure at each antenatal appointment. If your urine contains high levels of protein, and/or you have high blood pressure, you will be referred to the hospital for further tests.

The exact cause of pre-eclampsia is not fully understood, but it is believed to be related to abnormalities within the placenta, which supplies nutrients and oxygen to the baby. Factors that may increase the risk of developing pre-eclampsia include:

— first-time pregnancy

— being under 20 or over 40 years of age

— being overweight or obese before pregnancy

— carrying twins or triplets

— existing health conditions, such as chronic hypertension, diabetes, kidney disease and certain autoimmune disorders

— ethnicity – Black women of African and Caribbean descent have a higher risk. Five X More discuss a few of the reasons behind this further on page 74.

Pre-eclampsia can have serious consequences for both the mother and the baby if left untreated. Complications of pre-eclampsia may include:

— **Eclampsia:** Severe pre-eclampsia can progress to eclampsia, leading to seizures or convulsions, which can be life-threatening.

— **HELLP syndrome:** A rare but serious complication of pre-eclampsia that involves haemolysis (destruction of red blood cells), elevated liver enzymes and low platelet count, which can lead to liver failure, bleeding problems and organ damage.

— **Premature birth:** Pre-eclampsia increases the risk of premature birth, which can result in complications for the baby, including respiratory distress syndrome, jaundice and developmental delays.

The management of pre-eclampsia depends on the severity of the condition and the gestational age of the baby. Treatment options may include regular monitoring of blood pressure, urine protein levels and foetal wellbeing through ultrasound scans and foetal heart-rate monitoring. Blood-pressure-lowering medications, such as antihypertensives, may be prescribed to manage hypertension and prevent complications.

In severe cases of pre-eclampsia, hospitalisation may be necessary for close monitoring and management of complications until symptoms improve or the baby is born.

The only cure for pre-eclampsia is the birth of the baby and placenta. In some cases, an induction of labour or caesarean may be recommended if the risks of remaining pregnant outweigh the risks of the baby being born. Sometimes symptoms of pre-eclampsia are present postnatally, so any of the following signs should be reported: severe headaches, chest pain, sudden swelling of the face, hands and feet, visual disturbances, and generally not feeling quite right.

GESTATIONAL DIABETES

Gestational diabetes mellitus (GDM) is a form of diabetes that develops during pregnancy, typically in the second or third trimester. It causes high blood sugar levels that can be harmful to both mother and baby if left untreated. Unlike type 1 or 2 diabetes, GDM usually fully resolves after the baby has been born.

Several factors increase the likelihood of developing gestational diabetes. These include increased maternal age, a family history of diabetes, obesity, polycystic ovary syndrome (PCOS), previous gestational diabetes, and a history of delivering large babies or stillbirths. Ethnicity also plays a role, with women of African, Middle Eastern, Indigenous American, Mediterranean and South Asian descent being more

prone to gestational diabetes. If you are thought to be in a higher-risk category, you will be offered a glucose tolerance test (GTT) at around 26 to 28 weeks' gestation.

Sometimes medication is needed to regulate sugar levels, but often, changes to the diet can help to control it. A diabetic specialist midwife will support you if you have GDM.

Women with gestational diabetes are usually offered an induction if they haven't gone into labour spontaneously by 41 weeks. Occasionally it is offered earlier if there are any additional factors, such as high blood pressure, or if the diabetes is not under control through a healthy diet and appropriate medication.

ICP

Intrahepatic cholestasis of pregnancy (ICP) is a liver disorder characterised by reduced bile flow, leading to a build-up of bile acids in the bloodstream. This condition typically manifests in the third trimester and may recur in subsequent pregnancies.

The build-up of bile acids can cause intense itching, particularly on the hands and feet, which is why you should always mention any itching to your midwife, though itching during pregnancy doesn't always indicate a problem, as it's common in the third trimester due to stretching skin. Other signs and symptoms of ICP include dark urine and pale stools. If ICP is suspected, liver-function blood tests may be recommended.

Treatment may include medication to reduce bile acids and alleviate itching. Regular monitoring of foetal wellbeing may also be advised. Induction of labour may be recommended before full term to minimise complications, such as foetal distress or stillbirth.

Risk factors for obstetric cholestasis include a family history of the condition, multiple pregnancies and a personal history of liver disease.

PLACENTA PRAEVIA

The placenta usually embeds in the upper part of the uterus after conception, but with a placenta praevia, it implants lower down – either close to the cervix, or covering or partially covering it.

This abnormal positioning can be problematic, particularly during labour and birth. The baby needs to exit through the cervix during a vaginal birth and if the placenta is completely covering it, this is not an option.

Placenta praevia is often classified into different grades based on the extent of coverage over the cervix.

— **Grade 1** – placenta being within 2cm of the cervix but not covering it (also known as a low-lying placenta)

— **Grade 2** – partial coverage

— **Grade 3** – almost complete coverage

— **Grade 4** – the placenta is completely covering the cervix

The type of placenta praevia influences the management and treatment options, as more significant coverage increases the risk of complications.

Painless vaginal bleeding is one of the many signs and symptoms of placenta praevia, and it is especially common in the later stages of pregnancy. Nevertheless, not every case has symptoms that are apparent, and regular ultrasound is frequently used to make the diagnosis. A follow-up ultrasound is typically recommended later in pregnancy if a placenta is found to be low lying, to assess its proximity to the cervix. Many women who have been told they have a low-lying placenta at the 20-week scan will find that it is further away from the cervix at a later ultrasound. This is not because the placenta has moved, but rather that the stretching uterus has made the gap between the cervix and placenta longer.

A placenta praevia may result in heavy bleeding, the need for a caesarean section and preterm birth. Since there is a higher chance of excessive bleeding during labour and birth, if you are diagnosed with a placenta praevia, your care provider will work with you to devise a birth plan that is safest for you and your baby. A caesarean is recommended for placenta praevia at around 36 to 39 weeks. If the placenta is lying low, but is more than 2cm from the cervix, there is the option for a vaginal birth. If heavy bleeding occurs during pregnancy, a caesarean might be recommended earlier than 36 weeks.

Placenta praevia is more likely to develop if risk factors are present. These include pregnancy with multiples (such as twins or triplets), an advanced maternal age, previous caesarean sections and a history of uterine surgery. Additionally, there may be an increased risk for pregnant women who smoke or take cocaine.

GROUP B STREP

You may or may not have heard about group B streptococcus (GBS). It's a bacterium, also known as *Streptococcus agalactiae*, and is commonly found in the intestines, rectum and vagina of healthy adults without causing any symptoms. GBS can occasionally cause infections in newborn babies if transmitted during the birth, which can cause complications. Premature babies are at higher risk of developing issues as a result of GBS because their bodies and immune systems aren't sufficiently developed to fight off infections. If GBS is identified during pregnancy, antibiotics are usually offered during labour. If antibiotics aren't given for any reason, such as the birth occurred quickly before there was time to administer them, it may be recommended that the baby receives them instead.

GBS is not routinely tested for in the UK, and the UK National Screening Committee gives several reasons for this. A large number of people carry GBS, and the majority of those will give birth to babies that won't go on to develop an infection. Based on this, screening everyone in late pregnancy will not accurately predict which babies will go on to develop an infection. The optimal time for the test to be carried out is between 35 and 37 weeks, which would be too late for the babies most at risk of serious complications – premature ones. The Committee argues that giving antibiotics to everyone who has a positive GBS test would result in an extremely large number of women being given antibiotics that they do not need. Also, GBS can sometimes be detected in pregnancy but test negative during labour – which results in people who should be having antibiotics not receiving them.

So how is GBS detected? It's sometimes identified during pregnancy through vaginal swabs and urine tests that are carried out for other reasons. In these cases, antibiotics during labour are offered. This does create a problem for those who don't have any swabs or urine samples sent to the lab and then go on to pass GBS on to their babies unknowingly during labour, as they are not given antibiotics, and those infants subsequently develop infections.

Some parents may be anxious about whether or not they carry GBS. This can be even more worrying for them if they know someone whose baby developed severe complications as a result.

For any parents wishing to take a test in pregnancy, they can be done if paid for privately. More information can be found at Group B Strep Support (gbss.org.uk).

YOUR STORIES

'I tested positive for gestational diabetes in my second and third pregnancies.' — Karen

While thankfully the diabetes did not appear to impact either of my babies in terms of potential complications, the impact on me and my emotional wellbeing was huge. The information provided by the NHS was, in my view, outdated. Luckily I am somebody who researches (knowledge is power!) and I found lots of helpful information online which I put into practice in terms of the new diet. It's a huge responsibility – eating right, testing blood sugars four times a day, extra appointments/scans, anxiety, baby having blood sugars tested after birth. Yet people still minimise it and there is an undertone of it being lifestyle-related. I am within a healthy weight range and eat well and I still got it. I followed the diet without exception in both pregnancies and still needed the medication to stabilise my blood sugars. It was a lot. And I wish more people knew about it as it was very isolating.

Davina: Karen, I love the fact that you talk about doing your own research. When something happens to you in pregnancy, it is really important that you look everywhere for information in all the correct places. But it's great that you also took care of yourself in terms of your diet. So well done, and I'm pleased everything was fine with your births.

YOUR STORIES

'At 19 days old, our beautiful baby girl Mia lost her battle with meningitis, which resulted from a group B strep (GBS) infection.' — Amy

It is thought that Mia came into contact with GBS during delivery. We hadn't been made aware of GBS and its risks in my pregnancy, despite Royal College of Obstetricians and Gynaecologists (RCOG) guidance that expectant mothers should be given a leaflet. I believe that all expectant parents should be given knowledge that empowers them to make informed choices. A positive GBS test result does not need to lead to a negative outcome, but knowing that you are positive can ensure you get the right care and monitoring during your labour. I am still working with our hospital to bring about change and ensure other families don't end up in our situation. I have gone on to birth a healthy baby boy; Mia will always be with us.

Davina: Oh, Amy, your story broke my heart. This is why talking about birth and giving parents-to-be more information is so vital – so that we can be armed with the knowledge we need and feel empowered to ask for the care we deserve when we feel we're not being given it. Thank you for sharing your story, which I hope will help to encourage other parents to speak out so that we can prevent tragedies like yours happening again.

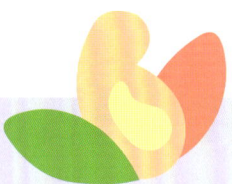

COLOSTRUM HARVESTING

Midwife Marley

Colostrum harvesting is a term we use when referring to the process of collecting and storing the first milk produced by breasts during late pregnancy. Doing this is not essential, but it has several benefits for both mothers and babies.

Colostrum starts developing in the breasts from around 16 weeks' gestation and continues until a few days after birth when the milk changes, increasing in volume. Some women will find that they leak colostrum during pregnancy, and others won't. I have had many conversations with women who are worried that not leaking milk during pregnancy means they won't have any milk. It doesn't! Colostrum comes in very small quantities, but is rich in nutrients, providing essential nourishment for the first few days of a baby's life.

Gaining familiarity with your breasts and how they function by expressing milk and harvesting colostrum during pregnancy will boost your confidence when it comes to breastfeeding. It can also be helpful if you are unable to feed your newborn right away.

Colostrum harvesting may also be beneficial to women who:

— have pre-existing or gestational diabetes (see page 146)

— have multiple sclerosis or breast hypoplasia (underdeveloped breast tissue not producing milk)

— are having a planned caesarean section

— have a history of breast surgery

— take certain high-blood-pressure medications during pregnancy

— have a strong family history of inflammatory bowel disease

— have had trouble breastfeeding after previous pregnancies

— are expecting more than one baby

— have a body mass index (BMI) score of 35 or above

— have a hormonal condition like polycystic ovary syndrome (PCOS)

If a baby has a known congenital condition or it's likely that they will spend some time in the NICU, colostrum harvesting may be of benefit.

For those who decide to harvest colostrum, it's recommended to begin after 36 weeks. Some people may worry that doing so could trigger labour, but this is highly unlikely. That said, it's advised not to express colostrum before birth if you:

— have placenta praevia

— have a history of preterm labour

— have a cervical stitch in place

If in doubt, speak with your midwife or obstetric doctor.

The best way to express colostrum for harvesting is by hand. As the quantities are extremely low (a few drops at a time), the colostrum would get lost within a breast pump. Hand expressing is more effective with the use of a syringe or cup. You can purchase colostrum-harvesting kits online or ask your infant-feeding team at the hospital to see if they have any available. A video demonstrating hand expressing is available on my YouTube and Instagram channels (@midwifemarley).

To hand express:

— **Step 1:** Wash your hands thoroughly with soap and warm water. Gently massage the breasts to stimulate milk flow.

— **Step 2:** Place the thumb and fingers around the breast, just behind the areola, in a 'C' shape with the thumb above.

— **Step 3:** Press gently inwards towards the chest wall and then compress and release the breast tissue rhythmically to express colostrum into a sterile container (from a colostrum-harvesting kit, or use a small container placed in a bottle steriliser).

— **Step 4:** Use a syringe to withdraw the colostrum from the container, place the syringe in a zip-lock bag, then in the freezer for storage. It can remain there for up to six months if the freezer is set to −18°C or lower. Make sure it's labelled with the date and time of expression.

PERINEAL MASSAGE

I felt really engaged in my pregnancies and wanted to do everything I could to prepare physically for the birth and support my body through that time, and as I've said, I was particularly nervous about tearing. That meant I was all in on anything I could do to help reduce the chances of tearing – and one option was perineal massage. As Marley explains, there's evidence to show that it can reduce your risk of tears – particularly the advanced kind – so if you're physically able to give it a go, I'd highly recommend it.

Marley: Perineal massage is a technique you can carry out during the last few weeks of pregnancy to help prepare the perineum (the area between the vagina and the anus) for childbirth. By gently stretching and massaging the perineal tissues, perineal massage aims to increase the flexibility and elasticity of the area.

Several studies have found evidence supporting the effectiveness of perineal massage in reducing the risk of perineal tearing during childbirth. One review of evidence concluded that perineal massage during the last month of pregnancy reduced the likelihood of serious perineal trauma requiring suturing or episiotomy (see page 195).

The technique is recommended by many midwives and maternity services. It is most effective when done two to three times per week, from 36 weeks' gestation, and only takes a few minutes. With a big bump, perineal massage isn't always easy to do by yourself. If you find it difficult, you could always ask your partner for help.

I have created a video demonstrating how to carry out a perineal massage on both Instagram and YouTube if you are a visual learner, but for now, here are the step-by-step instructions. You will need a lubricating oil such as grapeseed or olive oil.

— **Step 1:** Find a quiet space where you have full privacy and ensure you have clean hands.

— **Step 2:** Get into a comfortable position, ensuring your legs are spread wide and your knees are bent. You may find that propping a foot on the toilet or side of the bath helps if you are attempting to do it by yourself.

— **Step 3:** Place your thumbs just within the wall either side of your vagina. Your thumbs should only enter a couple of centimetres or so. If you find it easier, using a mirror might help you to see.

— **Step 4:** Using your thumbs, apply pressure to the sides and towards your anus. You will feel a stretching sensation but it shouldn't hurt. If it starts to hurt, stop and try again with less pressure. Hold this position for a minute.

— **Step 5:** Now move your thumbs slightly up and downwards towards the perineum, massaging the area in a 'U' shape. Continue to do this for a couple of minutes.

There are some circumstances in which perineal massage is not recommended, including for those who have been diagnosed with placenta praevia, or have an infection on the hands or fingers, vaginal thrush or any other open wounds in the perineal or vaginal area.

Braxton Hicks contractions are a normal and natural part of pregnancy, and they serve as a way for the uterus to prepare for labour.

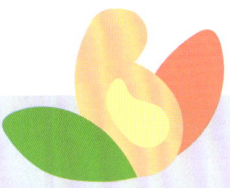

BRAXTON HICKS

Midwife Marley

At some point during your pregnancy, you might feel your belly go hard for a few seconds and even change into an odd, pointed shape. If this happens, it's likely to be a Braxton Hicks contraction. These are often referred to as 'practice contractions'; they are sporadic and irregular uterine contractions that occur during pregnancy, typically in the second and third trimesters. They are painless, though sometimes uncomfortable tightenings that can happen several times a day, but they are not harmful. Everyone will have them, but not everyone notices them.

Braxton Hicks contractions are a normal and natural part of pregnancy, and they serve as a way for the uterus to prepare for labour. However, if you experience frequent or painful contractions that persist or increase in intensity, it's essential to contact your maternity unit for guidance and to rule out preterm labour (see page 157). Braxton Hicks contractions may become annoying and uncomfortable, particularly if they happen frequently. To manage them and alleviate discomfort, you can try the following:

— **Change positions:** Sometimes, a change in position, such as lying down on your left side or taking a warm bath, can help relieve Braxton Hicks contractions.

— **Stay hydrated:** Dehydration can trigger or exacerbate Braxton Hicks contractions, so it's essential to drink plenty of water throughout the day.

— **Practise relaxation techniques:** Deep-breathing exercises, relaxation techniques or gentle massages may help relax the uterine muscles and reduce the intensity of the contractions.

— **Empty your bladder:** A full bladder can irritate the uterus and trigger the tightenings, so make sure to empty your bladder regularly.

— **Rest:** Sometimes, fatigue or overexertion can contribute to Braxton Hicks contractions, so it's important to listen to your body and rest when needed.

I got really excited when I could feel Braxton Hicks. In fact, I was so excited – because I thought real labour had started – that I didn't go to sleep. Big mistake, as I was of course exhausted the next day. The other interesting thing is that if you do try to go to sleep when you've got Braxton Hicks – which I strongly suggest you do – often they will stop. And if they turn into true labour, they will wake you up. I mean, nobody's ever slept through giving birth, so don't worry – your body will get you up and out of bed in order for you to birth your baby.

If contractions turn into true labour, they will wake you up.

I mean, nobody's ever slept through giving birth, so don't worry – your body will get you up and out of bed in order for you to birth your baby.

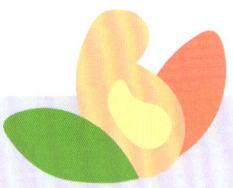

PRETERM LABOUR

Midwife Marley

Sometimes babies will make an appearance much earlier than anticipated. Preterm labour is one that begins before 37 weeks' gestation. Babies need at least 37 weeks in the uterus to develop and grow, but spontaneous labour can begin before this for a number of reasons, many of which can be complex and multifactorial. They may include persistent urinary tract infections, abdominal trauma, maternal health conditions, such as diabetes and high blood pressure, or a weakened cervix. Additionally, multiple pregnancies and certain lifestyle factors, such as smoking and drug use, are linked to an increased likelihood of preterm labour.

The gestational age at which preterm babies are born has a significant impact on their prognosis. The closer the birth comes to full term, the better they are likely to do. Extremely preterm babies born before 28 weeks of gestation have a far greater chance of developing complications than babies born between 32 and 37 weeks.

Depending on the gestational age of the pregnancy, medical therapies for preterm labour may involve the use of drugs such as tocolytics, which temporarily decrease contractions to delay labour. In order to decrease the risk of respiratory distress syndrome and hasten the development of the baby's lungs, corticosteroids may also be given. This is because the baby's lungs are not fully developed until around 37 weeks. Maternity hospitals in the UK will have neonatal intensive-care units attached that are fully prepared to care for babies in the event of a preterm birth.

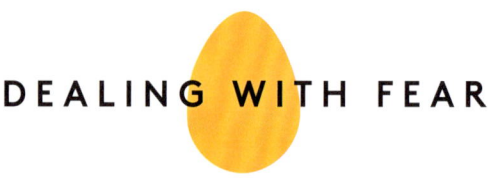

DEALING WITH FEAR

For me, the best way to combat fear and anxiety around pregnancy and labour is to be prepared. To learn about everything; to make sure that you have every eventuality covered; to make sure that you are in the best position possible to be as happy and calm and present as you have ever been in your life. I don't think I really understood the meaning of being present until it happened to me for the first time very recently. And it happened during a breathing class. This concept of being in the moment, and not thinking about tomorrow, or what I'm going to do at the end of the week, or what I did yesterday, but actually just thinking about the breath that I'm taking and just lying there, is so liberating for your mind and your body. I cannot recommend using breathing techniques enough to combat feelings of anxiety and worrying about the future.

We've talked about a birth plan and how important that is (see page 91), but going to see the hospital, meeting the midwives, talking to them and asking questions – all of these kinds of things are going to make you feel less nervous about labour because you know what the place looks like, and you can picture the people you're going to be meeting. It's said that knowledge is power, but knowledge can also be a reliever of stress: not knowing things, not knowing where you're going, and being a bit scared because of those unknowns, is the opposite of what you want. So get as much knowledge as you possibly can.

When I was pregnant there were moments when I felt like I'd lost any control I had over my body and mind, as if I'd literally been taken over by another human being, so it's really nice when you say to yourself, 'Right, I am going to take control of this. And I am going to learn as much as I can. And make sure that I enter this experience empowered by knowledge.'

I remember finding much of the language around labour very unhelpful. That's why I like to call contractions 'rushes'. I learned that from American midwife and author Ina May Gaskin – she calls them rushes, and I thought that was a much nicer word than 'contraction'. A contraction sounds painful. A rush sounds quite exciting. These things matter. Words matter because they are extremely powerful. The person who really transformed my thinking around this was the therapist and author Marisa Peer. She talks about words shaping our reality and how we have the power to make ourselves feel much better – or worse – with the words we use around our labour.

Let's take the word 'pain', for example. I think the thing that causes expectant mothers the most fear is the idea of pain – that labour and birth are going to really hurt. Pain is normally something that would be frightening, because it occurs when something bad is happening, like we've fallen over or been in an accident. But the pain your rushes are going to cause will be bringing you closer to meeting your baby. And you only have a finite number of rushes to get through before you meet them. So it's almost like you need to have a word with that intense feeling that comes with a rush and you go, 'Bring it on, give me the most intense rushes you can. Because they are going to bring this life that I've been growing for nine months into my arms.'

The other thing to remember is that labour pain is safe pain. It is not pain to be feared. My mantra was, 'It's safe to open even more.' I kept repeating it. So you just need to keep yourself loose, keep yourself relaxed. I think the reason I loved giving birth was because I became very animal. I really had to go inside myself and listen to my instincts – my gut instincts – and they knew what to do. I was braver than I'd ever been before. I looked fear right in the eye and I went, 'You're going to be okay, this is safe pain.'

I can't lie to you – it is really intense. But when you have delivered a baby, you will have done an amazing thing, and that's something to be incredibly proud of.

Another thing that really, really helped me deal with the fear was that Ina May

Gaskin's book told me to keep my sense of humour, in it she says: 'If you can't be a hero, you can at least be funny while being a chicken.' And I love that, because it's true; sometimes you might feel in such pain and want to scream, but then something will happen, and you'll be able to make a joke or somebody else will make a joke, and you will laugh with them instead of wanting to throw everything at them.

Remember, everybody who is in this birth with you is looking at you; you are the central force of energy in your labour and if you're frightened or angry, it puts everybody in the room in a stressed state. But if you're relaxed, and you smile and you laugh (I know that is a brave and difficult thing to do), you can find a way of comforting yourself through this, which I know you can do. You need to find a way of talking to yourself that helps soothe you. Mine was mantras; breathing; informing myself. What will help you? Really think about it. Don't start thinking about it two, three weeks before you give birth. Think about it now. Be on it – you'll feel proud of yourself for that, too. The more organised you are, the less stressful it will be. You might not feel like you know what to do. But you know what to do.

My mantra was, 'It's safe to open even more.' I kept repeating it.

COPING WITH FEAR

Dr Caroline Boyd, Perinatal Clinical Psychologist and Author

Through all the uncertainty around birth, you may feel intense waves of fear. Just as you'll experience strong physical 'rushes' in labour, you may notice emotional 'rushes' as you worry about your baby's health or how you'll cope in labour. Some degree of fear and anxiety is completely normal – it's part of the process of birthing and becoming a parent. The task is not getting rid of the fear but to try to stay open to events as they unfold and work with fear as it arises.

Understanding how fear shows up in our brain and body is key. Our tricky 'emotional' brain is hardwired to keep us safe. This means our threat system is highly sensitive and reactive. Birth can bring many new 'what if' worries about our baby's safety, fear around managing pain, or uncertainty linked to our birthing environment. Just as a life-or-death threat, such as a predatory attack, triggers our internal

alarm system, all these threats send the same 'danger!' signal – activating the fight, flight, freeze reaction in our sympathetic nervous system. Adrenaline and cortisol flood our body, preparing us for action. We breathe faster and our heart rate increases. In a highly fearful state, we shift into freeze mode (feeling paralysed), or appeasement (becoming submissive). These are simply our 'tricky' brain's way of protecting us.

Efforts to resist or avoid the fear are understandable. Yet fighting anxious thoughts or labelling ourselves 'bad' for having them only increases their power and intensity. Instead, mindfully direct attention to your breath or body to anchor yourself and find your internal place of safety. Next time you feel the cold grip of fear, name it to tame it. Notice and name your feelings with kindness and without judgment, then try to let any anxious thoughts go.

Tell yourself gently: 'I am feeling scared *and* I am safe.'

Ina May Gaskin's book told me to keep my sense of humour:

'If you can't be a hero, you can at least be funny while being a chicken.'

And I love that, because it's true; sometimes you might feel in such pain and want to scream, but then something will happen, and you'll be able to make a joke or somebody else will make a joke, and you will laugh with them instead of wanting to throw everything at them.

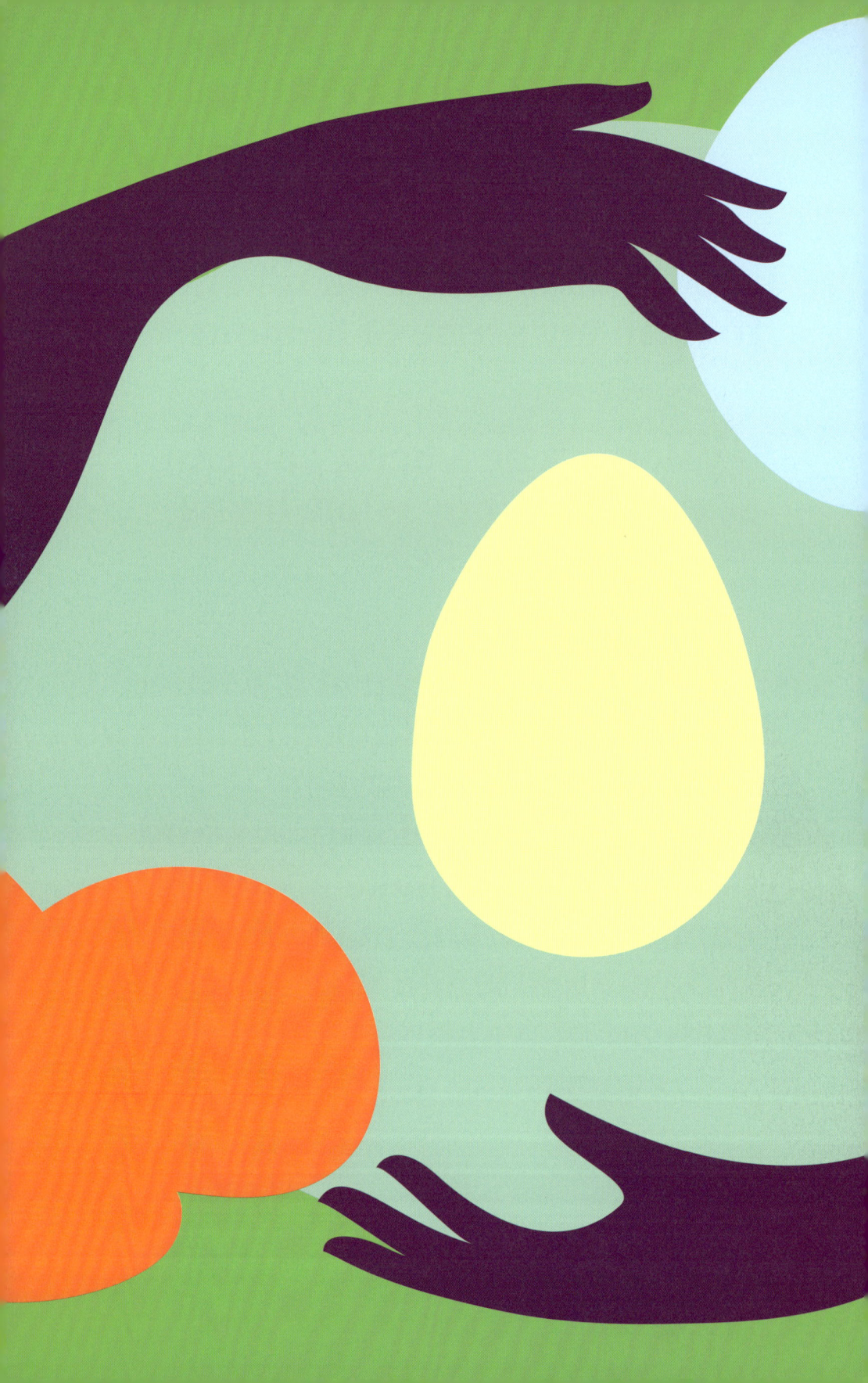

CHAPTER 5

BIRTH

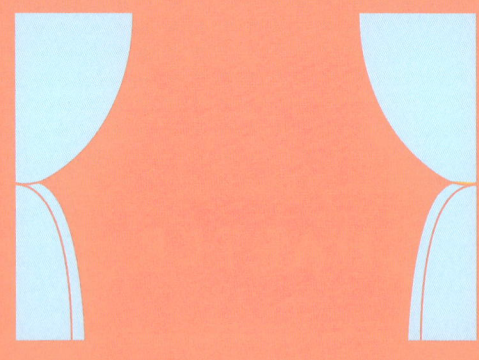

So, here are we are - the main event.

Read this again and again - and again, LONG before you get into that birthing room.

IT'S HAPPENING...

This chapter is the one I want you to read again and again – and again, LONG before you get into that birthing room. It will help inform the decisions you make about your birth plan and I hope it will help guide you through the many different means and ways to give birth, prepare you for the different scenarios that can arise, and empower you to make the decisions that will support the birthing experience that is right for you and your baby.

But while reading books and doing your research are, in my opinion, vital, no amount of knowledge can enable you to predict how you will react to this event and how it will unfold. It won't necessarily happen as you'd planned; you may change your mind about how much pain relief you want or the type of labour that suits you, or your mind might be changed for you by the way your baby presents itself. What I can guarantee you, however, is that birthing another tiny human will be one of the most life-altering, seemingly miraculous moments you will ever experience in your life, and I truly hope that you're able to look back and feel that it was a joyful one. I hope there are times – even if it's just for a fraction of a second as you reach for your baby's head as it crowns, make that final push or watch the cord being cut – when you can enjoy the process and be so proud of what you are achieving. Giving birth changed my life in more ways than I could have imagined, and I know how lucky I am to be able to look back at each experience with such pride and happiness. I truly wish the same for you.

CREATING THE BEST BIRTHING ATMOSPHERE FOR YOU

I realise that, for me, giving birth at home immediately enabled me to feel comfortable and cocooned, but you can recreate something homely in hospital, provided that you arrive with time to do this. Sometimes, you want to stay at home as long as possible, so you'll be going into the final stage of labour as you arrive. But if, for example, it's your first birth and you're in hospital for ages, it is possible to try to create an atmosphere that is calming and soothing. The most important thing to think about is what will help you feel as relaxed as possible, because this helps stimulate all the feel-good hormones that will help you have a smooth labour.

Music is a big one for me. I like kind of chill, calm music, but just make sure you've got a playlist on hand of whatever music helps relax you. If listening to

Metallica is your happy place, then put on Metallica. If humming to yourself and swaying backwards or forwards is your jam, then do that – do whatever it takes to make yourself feel comfortable. Remember that you could be in labour for 12, 24 or even 36 hours, and you don't want to have to listen to your one-hour playlist 24 times – it'll drive you mad – so try to come up with a 12-hour playlist of mellow tunes. I have found (I'm not sponsored by them) Spotify to be the best for making playlists, as they offer lots of really good suggestions, but use any streaming platform you want.

Another way of creating a really nice atmosphere, for me, was lighting. I found I instinctively wanted to go into the warmest, darkest, quietest, safest place to give birth. Think of animals – they go off somewhere quiet, dark and safe when they give birth, and that was exactly what I wanted to do. With Holly, I went into the dog's room, and I was in a small room with a birthing pool with Tilly and Chester. You just really want to be somewhere calm and private, so the lighting needs to be dim and peaceful. If you are giving birth in a hospital and lighting is important to you, then hopefully you will have spoken to them about whether you can adjust it.

If you have an anxious partner, it might be you doing all the reassuring during labour, but the biggest thing you can do for your partner or birth partner to create a good atmosphere when you're giving birth is to tell them what to do. It is very reassuring for a birth partner to know what is helpful for you and what is not. For example, sometimes being asked repeatedly what you want can be quite annoying, so just tell them gently that if you need something, you'll let them know.

In her book *Spiritual Midwifery* (1975), Ina May Gaskin reminds us to be nice to the people around us. Remember to say please and thank you. Remember to look at them. I know that sometimes you will be so in the zone that this will be difficult, but just doing those small things for the people caring for you, which includes midwives, doctors, cleaning staff, your partner, friends, will help set the tone for a gentler, calmer atmosphere. If you're screaming at someone or swearing a lot, it makes everybody in the room tense. That will make you tense. And that's not what you want, as you might unwittingly suppress the magical hormone oxytocin, which is what facilitates the birth process.

Feeling as relaxed as possible helps stimulate the feel-good hormones that will help you have a smooth labour.

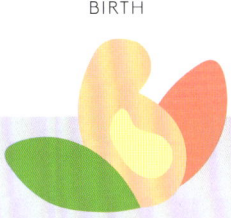

EARLY SIGNS OF LABOUR

Midwife Marley

The way labour begins varies from person to person, as do the signs of labour. While some women will have obvious signs leading up to the start of labour, some won't. Signs may begin in the days or hours leading up to its onset as the hormones change and the body starts to prepare the uterus. Here are a few indicators that labour could be on its way.

1. NESTING

As Davina has described, some women report a phenomenon known as 'nesting' (see page 136), in which, usually in the final hours or days before giving birth, they feel an inexplicable urge to make sure everything is ready for the new baby. They can find themselves doing chores they would never normally do, such as a thorough clean of the entire house or repeatedly washing and ironing the baby's clothes. Some women have spoken about having a strange feeling that they were going to go into labour right before they did! It's like an instinct – a bizarre feeling that you can't quite make sense of.

You may feel that you need to stay at home or get an overwhelming feeling that you don't want your partner to go to work that day 'just in case'.

2. LACK OF APPETITE

The digestive system slows down when you go into labour, as all the body's energy is required for the uterus to work efficiently. You may find that a sudden reduction in appetite could mean you are going into labour.

3. LOOSE BOWEL MOVEMENTS

If you are around your due date and you haven't eaten anything that could be upsetting your stomach, loose bowel movements could be a sign that labour is on its way.

4. MILD CRAMP-LIKE PAIN IN YOUR LOWER ABDOMEN OR BACK

Even though these cramps are somewhat typical during pregnancy, they may become more frequent in the final stages and once early labour has started. It's unlikely to be actual labour if you've been experiencing intermittent, mild pains that don't get progressively worse over the course of the day.

5. LOSS OF THE MUCUS PLUG

Losing the mucus plug is a common sign that labour may be approaching. This is a thick, gel-like substance that seals the cervix during pregnancy, protecting the uterus from infection. As the cervix begins to soften, thin out (efface) and dilate in preparation for childbirth, the mucus plug may be expelled from the vagina. It is clear and jelly-like in texture. Occasionally it may have a brownish appearance due to old blood from the cervix. The mucus plug may come away in bits over the course of a few days, or in one piece. In many cases, women won't notice it coming away at all until they are in active labour.

If you do lose your mucus plug, labour is likely, but not certain, to begin within a couple of weeks. The terms 'mucus plug' and 'bloody show' are often used interchangeably but they are different things. While the plug is like a lump of jelly, a bloody show is mucus tinged with blood that is more like discharge. It usually occurs around or after the onset of labour as the cervix starts to make more rapid changes.

If you lose any mucus from the vagina that is green, bright red or offensive smelling, at any stage in pregnancy, contact your maternity team, as it may indicate an infection or other concern.

6. WATERS BREAKING (MEMBRANE RUPTURE)

Sometimes the bag of water surrounding the baby, known as the membrane sac, ruptures before labour begins. This only happens in around 10 per cent of cases, as most will break during labour. Some won't break at all, and the baby is born in the sac. This is called an 'en caul' birth, a Latin term. If a baby is born in the sac, the midwife or parents will gently pull the membranes away from the baby with their hands, at which point the baby takes their first breath.

For around 60 per cent of women, labour will begin within 24 hours of their waters breaking and for 96 per cent within four days. When the membranes are intact throughout pregnancy, there is a 0.5 per cent chance of developing an infection within the uterus. When the membranes have ruptured for more than 24 hours, this chance increases slightly to 1 per cent. For this reason, UK guidelines recommend offering labour induction after this time period. Not everyone will go ahead with an induction, however; some will decide to wait until the body goes into labour naturally while keeping an eye on their temperature and the baby's wellbeing with the support of their maternity team. Induction of labour will be discussed further on in the book to help support you in making informed decisions (see page 197). If your waters break and the fluid is green, red or brown, contact your maternity unit for further advice.

OXYTOCIN

Oxytocin is a hormone produced by the brain. It's called the 'love hormone': our bodies produce it when we fall in love, and it is released during sex, orgasm, birth and breastfeeding. During labour, if you're having a vaginal birth, its main function is to stimulate the muscles in the uterus to bring on contractions. You'll also get a surge of oxytocin in the final stage of labour, so it will help you with the pushing. Oxytocin has also been proven to reduce stress, so it calms you down and helps you deal with the pain during labour, while low oxytocin levels have been linked to depression and low mood, including postpartum depression. It's particularly important after the birth – you get a surge of it when you have skin-to-skin contact with your baby, helping you feel more relaxed and bonded with them. It also helps with the let-down reflex during breastfeeding by moving the milk from the ducts in the breast to the nipple.

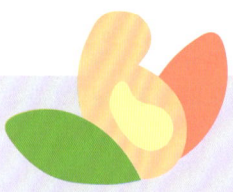

FALSE LABOUR

Midwife Marley

'False labour' refers to the frequent but irregular contractions some women may feel in the final few weeks of pregnancy. Although the term is used a lot, I don't really like to use it, as while the contractions may not be true labour contractions that result in the imminent birth of a baby, they are certainly helping things along! I prefer the term pre-labour or prodromal labour.

These contractions occur either in the abdomen or back, and may feel like period pains. They vary in length, frequency and intensity. Sometimes, they can come and go every 5, 10, 20 minutes or so over several hours before stopping. They then might start up again the following day. Although they may feel uncomfortable, they don't change in intensity or length, and don't follow any particular pattern for very long. Because of this, these contractions don't make any changes to the cervix significant enough to be classed as established labour.

I remember being told I was in false labour. With Holly, I woke up with contractions in the night and started timing them and they were a little bit all over the place. But they were definitely contractions. So I stayed up all night – I was so excited – and left my husband to sleep. And in the morning I said, 'I think I'm in labour.' So we called Caroline and she came. And when she examined me, she said, 'I've got to be honest with you, you're not dilated at all, you're in false labour and this could go on for days, so try to rest and sleep.' But I was so disheartened and frustrated that I went through another whole night trying to sleep with contractions coming and going. And when I woke up the next morning, I was still not dilated at all. But then Caroline measured me again six hours later, and I thought, *I'm still in false labour* – nothing felt that different – but Caroline said, 'Oh, you're 7cm dilated, congratulations.' I'd gone from nothing to 7cm in six hours. If you do experience this, I feel for you. I know how frustrating false labour can be, but just try to think of it as part of your birth story and keep yourself calm and relaxed, ready for when labour does actually start.

A BIT OF MYTH BUSTING

There are so many different things we're told about birth, and they're not all entirely true, so I just want to address some of the most common myths and set the record straight for you.

CRAVINGS WILL TELL YOU YOUR BABY'S SEX:

Lots of people say that if you're craving salty and sour food, or proteins, you're having a boy. And if you want sugar, you're having a girl. But there's no evidence to suggest there's any link between pregnancy cravings and a baby's sex. However, there is some research that suggests sometimes a non-food craving (I used to chew sponges in the shower – not real sponges; I'm talking synthetic, coloured sponges) can indicate a nutrient deficiency or anaemia, so do have a look at that and reach out to your doctor to get it checked.

FIRST BABIES ARE ALWAYS LATE:

Actually, first babies are only 5 per cent more likely to be born after 40 weeks than other babies. But first babies are 2 per cent more likely than other babies to be born preterm (before 37 weeks). There are lots of women who stop work two weeks before their due date and imagine that they're going to have two weeks at home, but sometimes the baby does come sooner.

BREASTFEEDING COMES REALLY EASILY:

Everybody talks about breastfeeding being the most natural thing in the world and how it comes really easily after giving birth. Breastfeeding your baby is a really natural thing to do, but it's not always easy and it's quite dependent on the type of birth you've had. One myth says you've got to get your baby on your boob as soon as possible after you've given birth for it to learn how to latch on, but that wasn't the case for me (see page 218). For plenty of women, breastfeeding isn't straightforward or their preferred choice, and we'll talk about this more later on (see page 248).

YOU CAN'T GET PREGNANT WHILE YOU'RE BREASTFEEDING:

This is quite a mega one. I've heard a lot that you can't get pregnant while you're breastfeeding. You can. Breastfeeding can park your periods for a bit, but it doesn't mean that you can't get pregnant. (Fancy another one? Ha ha. In joke.) So, if you're ready for another child, that's fine. But if you don't want to have another straight away, be sure to talk to your doctor about contraception.

The three stages of labour

There are three stages of labour, though stage 1 is in fact two parts: a latent stage of labour (also called 'early' or 'prodromal' labour) and then established (or 'active') labour.

STAGE 1: LATENT

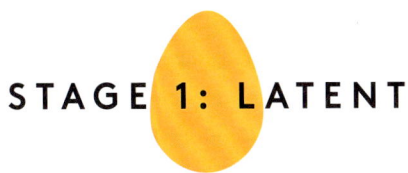

The latent phase is when your cervix starts to soften and dilate. You'll begin to experience contractions, which are starting to push your baby down into the birth canal and causing the cervix to open, ready for your baby to be born. This first stage will be made up of contractions that are irregular – they will get longer, stronger and more frequent, but the process can take hours (and, for some women, days).

The latent stage can be quite a confusing time. I would have moments where I would get contractions and think, *Oh, my goodness, this is labour*, but the contractions would be irregular and then I would lie down and they would suddenly stop. The contractions in the latent stage of labour can be slightly uncomfortable – a little niggle or even just a tightening.

Sometimes, your contractions will start thick and fast, and you'll go into established labour very quickly – if your contractions are coming regularly, it could possibly be the beginning of labour, so start timing them as soon as they start. I wrote down the timing between my contractions by hand because we didn't have apps in Holly's or Tilly's day, and that's a lovely keepsake (I've still got the pieces of paper in their memory boxes), but now you can track yours in an app – Storky, Freya and Contraction Timer have all been recommended to me as apps that are easy to use.

Sometimes your body plays tricks on you, and it isn't what you think – see the sections on Braxton Hicks contractions (page 155) and false labour (page 170). What's important to know is that when your contractions start, you will not have any idea how long or how fast your labour is going to be, so please consider your energy levels and your mental wellbeing and just try to stay comfortable and relaxed. Midwives often say that labour starts at night because it's a quiet time and we'll be free from distractions, and what's interesting is that all of mine did start at night. If it's your first labour, you will be so excited. I've yet to meet somebody who went back to bed when they started feeling contractions, but if you can, try to get some rest during this stage because if the contractions start in the evening, as mine did with Holly and Chester, there's a chance you're going to be up during the night. I know it's a very hard thing to do, but honestly, even with your first labour, try to go to sleep. It's worth remembering that no woman in the history of humankind has slept through giving birth. If your labour gets really intense, it will wake you up. Sleeping is not a representation of how long your birth is going to be – it's not going to slow your labour or make it longer. And if you can't sleep, make sure that you are eating snacks and drinking plenty of fluids, as these will help give you enough energy when you really need it. If you've learnt some breathing exercises, do them (see page 34).

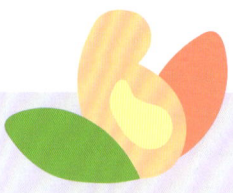

EATING AND DRINKING DURING LABOUR

Midwife Marley

Labour can be tiring, so eating and drinking during it can help keep your energy levels up and ensure your body remains hydrated, which is important for the uterus to contract effectively. In general, eating and drinking is considered safe during labour, although you may not feel like eating much, as nausea is common when you're experiencing contractions.

Having a squeezy sports bottle filled with water to hand throughout labour is a good way to ensure you have fluids ready and available. Water will help keep you hydrated, and isotonic drinks can help with energy and electrolyte balance. As well as sipping often, pee regularly, as keeping your bladder empty will help with the descent of the baby's head.

The best foods to eat during labour are small snacks that are high in complex carbs, proteins and other nutrients, rather than just sugary snacks like sweets and chocolate, which will offer you a quick lift but a sudden crash

afterwards. Fruits, nuts and cereal bars are all good options for providing you with a longer-lasting energy boost. You may want to add some tuna, or peanut butter sandwiches with wholemeal bread if you're feeling particularly hungry, but don't eat too fast! If you have any medications in labour, they can make you feel a little sick as your digestive system slows down. The best time to eat would be during early labour as it's likely you won't feel like eating much more as the labour progresses.

Eating may also not be advised if you receive opioids during labour (including epidurals), as it increases the risk of vomiting. If you have any of these types of analgesia and are feeling hungry, do discuss this with your midwife.

STAGE 1: ESTABLISHED

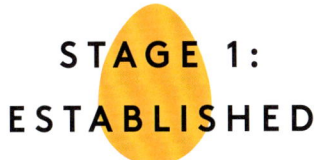

Marley: Established labour is defined as the point in which regular, strong contractions are experienced at least every four minutes, lasting 50 to 60 seconds for at least a couple of hours, in conjunction with a cervix that is dilated to around 3 to 4cm. As you likely won't know how much your cervix is dilating when you go into labour, keep an eye on the timing between contractions, as their intensity will help you determine when to call your midwife or maternity unit. You'll feel them get stronger over time and they will continue to do so until the birth. It's worth noting that if you have been practising hypnobirthing (see page 118), you'll probably appear a lot calmer externally, so do let your midwife know when your contractions intensify so that they don't assume you are simply in pre-labour!

WHEN TO MAKE THE CALL

So, when do you call your midwife? Below are a few indicators that it's time to pick up the phone:

— Your contractions are regular (about every five minutes or more frequently).

— Your waters break.

— You feel like you might need pain relief.

— You're worried about anything.

If you have any doubts or you think you're in labour and you're not sure what to do, please do just contact your maternity unit or midwife about your symptoms. They'll tell you what to do next.

If you go into hospital, be prepared for the fact that they might send you home again. I know lots of people who felt very deflated when they went in and were told to go home because they weren't very far along. I know that can feel so disappointing, but it is nice to be at home, so just hold on to that. If you do go home and then suddenly feel it's got a lot more intense, and you really think you are in labour, do listen to yourself.

Once you're in hospital and you are well dilated, you will get checked and offered pain relief if that's part of your birth plan. When I was in labour at home, Pam would check the baby and see how it was getting on because I wanted to be monitored. She would make sure she could hear the baby's heartbeat and give me guidance on positions and things like that.

I really wanted to walk around for most of the time, and sway my hips backwards and forwards. When I was having a contraction, I would not be able to talk to anybody, but I remember leaning on my kitchen work surface. And sometimes, without realising it, I would go onto my tiptoes when it got really intense. Pam would always say, 'You're on your tiptoes again.' And I would think, *God, am I?* and I would try to put my feet on the floor because Pam told me that when you're on your tiptoes, your bottom's clenching, and actually what you want to do is relax, not clench. It's the same with your mouth: if your mouth is tense, then your bottom and your cervix might be tense, too, so try to keep your mouth relaxed. Try to keep your body relaxed, try to breathe through the contractions. Just think about it being safe pain, letting yourself open, not trying to stop it or work against it. Go with it. Listen to yourself.

At this point your midwife will be thinking about your birth plan, so if you have requested an epidural, then this

is when your healthcare professional will be talking to you about this.

Your cervix needs to dilate to 10cm for your baby to be able to pass through it, and when it gets to that stage, it's fully dilated. Sometimes people get checked and will be 4cm, and the next time they get checked four hours later they will still be 4cm. I cannot tell you how disheartening, demotivating or disappointing that can feel. You start thinking, *Why am I not doing this right?* But that just isn't the case. There isn't a right or a wrong way to give birth. Sometimes, you might not dilate for four or five hours; sometimes people can go from nothing to 5cm in an hour. So please don't get disheartened by anything. You are where you're meant to be. Your labour is where it's meant to be, and you *will* get there.

In a first pregnancy, from the start of the established stage of labour to being fully dilated can last a long time – from 8 to 18 hours on average, but it was 24 hours for me with Holly, which is why I said to really try resting at the beginning.

TRANSITION

When you reach the end of the first stage of labour, this is when everything changes. By this point, your contractions – or rushes – will be quite close together, and very intense. When I was about to start pushing, I was always sent a sign. My body told me when I was transitioning to the next stage of labour by making me cry. Every time I would spontaneously cry, and I would never quite know why, it would just happen, and I would think, *Okay, I need to prep myself for the next* phase. It really is a miracle. And the other miracle is that whenever I went through a rush, I could feel it coming. It's like a wave – it builds and then it decreases. And so I could prepare myself by getting myself into a position where I could go through the rush. And just when I was thinking, *I can't do this anymore – this is too much, it's too intense*, the pain started subsiding. That is the miracle of labour because I was never given more pain than I could handle.

POOING
DURING LABOUR

Everybody kept telling me I was going to poo during labour, and one of the things that was slowing me down with Holly was that I was frightened of pooing. The midwife said to me, 'If you poo, we will be so proud of you, because we know you're pushing in the right way.' I know it can be a horrifying thought, but honestly, if you poo during labour and you've got midwives present, the poo will be there for about two and a half seconds – the midwives will just spirit it away (what poo?) and you'll move on.

STAGE 2: ACTIVE LABOUR

The second stage of labour lasts from when your cervix is fully dilated until your baby is born.

When I had Holly, I was told that I would just know when I needed to push. And I thought, *But how do you know?* What I find fascinating about the physiology of the body is that, if you haven't had an epidural, you will absolutely know when it is time to push because you do not push – your body begins to try to EXPEL the baby. That is the best way that I can describe it; it is not an action that you are taking. This is an action that your body appears to be doing all by itself.

The feeling, for me, started like a shudder in my muscles at the bottom of my stomach, which moved up over the baby to by my ribcage. And the shudder would kind of squeeze and contract my muscles in my stomach, to physically move the baby down the birth canal. I could feel it happening, but I would have been unable to stop a push. I could breathe through it and maybe make it bearable. And I could push at the same time as my body was expelling the baby and that would make the push more intense. But I couldn't have stopped it.

At this stage of your labour, your midwife will be helping you find a position to give birth in. A lot of women at this point are being monitored – maybe you've asked to be monitored; maybe the medical professionals with you want you to be monitored. It may be that there's been an issue of some sort and so the doctors or midwives want to keep you lying down; this means lots of women end up either sort of lying down or in a semi-sitting position when they give birth. This is completely fine. However, studies show that being in an upright position – standing, in a squat, or on your knees – makes the second stage of labour shorter because gravity helps pull the baby's head down towards the birth canal. There's also something about the angle of the head in your pelvis that is supported when you're squatting. I wanted to squat on the floor or kneel in the birthing pool to give birth – those were the positions I really wanted to get into. But find a position that feels comfortable and instinctive to you.

When you get to the pushing stage, if you're having your first baby, that shouldn't last more than three hours. At the end of three hours with Holly, Caroline looked at me and said, 'If you don't get this baby out in the next three pushes, we're going to hospital.' What I thought was amazing was that I was just so tired, I thought I had nothing left. But when she said that, I got Holly out in two pushes. I found the strength to do it. We all have the ability to be superhuman in labour.

If you were to ask me what the most intense part of labour is, I would say the same thing for each birth, and that is the crowning, which is when the baby's head is about to come out. The stinging and the intensity were a lot. But this is when midwives are wonderful because they can see what's happening and they just get you to breathe, to slow everything down a bit, because what you really want to do is let your baby's head be born slowly and gently. The reason why it stings so much is because your skin is trying to stretch to make space for the head to come out. And you want to give your vagina and anus and perineum time to stretch, which means there is less likelihood of tearing (see page 194).

So, the midwife will tell you what to do when the baby's head is about to come out. At this point, it's quite intense, but you are so close to meeting your baby. And once your baby's head has come out, really the hard work is over because the rest of the body will usually be born with the next rush. Every time I had a baby, the body followed with the next rush, but sometimes it might take two rushes.

If you've had your baby lying down, it will be placed on your chest. If you've given birth in the water, you will scoop your baby out between your legs and into your arms. When I gave birth squatting, that was quite funny because my dog was the first person to say hello to Holly when she was on the floor and I just scooped her up.

YOUR STORIES

'I was in labour for my second birth at home and when I started contractions, I went into my bedroom and just wanted to be left alone.' — Jacqui

I was not afraid, but felt I needed to be away somewhere quiet and safe. Once my contractions got pretty close together, I went through into the kitchen, stopping for each contraction, and told my husband, who was batch-cooking food, that we needed to call the midwife and fill the pool. It all felt very matter-of-fact. The funny part of my home birth was delivering the placenta, which took a lot more time. I had to get out of the pool, and ended up giving birth to the

placenta on the toilet – a good position for me but less convenient for the midwife!

Davina: Thank you, Jacqui. Where we choose to give birth is funny, isn't it? I totally understand that feeling of wanting to go and labour on your own. It's a time to concentrate and listen to your body and if you're in a quiet space, you can listen to your instincts – they will tell you what positions to get into.

STAGE 3:
PLACENTAL DELIVERY

The third stage of labour is the one I feel no one told me about. Or, if they did, I actively chose to ignore it, because I gave birth to Holly and I remember thinking afterwards, *What's going on?* and then being told I still had to give birth to the placenta!

There are two different ways to manage this stage of labour: one is physiological, and one is managed. Marley is going to talk you through each one below, but essentially, which route you go down will be a conversation to have with your midwife. I just let the placenta come out when it was ready, which was about 40 minutes after each baby. Interestingly, the second and third time I birthed the placenta, it was more painful than the first; with Chester it was actually quite intense. It's a bit like giving birth all over again – I mean, obviously it doesn't go on for as long, but it was quite painful. So, knowing what I knew after Holly's birth, after I gave birth to Tilly and Chester, I immediately took a couple of paracetamols just to get me through the birthing of the placenta, and that helped.

Nowadays people don't cut the umbilical cord straight away; it's generally left to pulse for a bit so that blood can flow back to the baby, which increases the amount of iron and other nutrients they receive. Marley will also talk you through more of the benefits of delaying the cord clamping and cutting, on page 182.

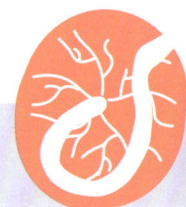

BIRTHING THE PLACENTA

Marley: Once the baby has been born, you'll probably be feeling relief and joy, but it's not quite over yet. The third stage of labour refers to the period after the baby has been born and ends when the placenta and foetal membranes leave your body. The uterus will begin to contract again soon after the birth to help the placenta come away. Sometimes this is as soon as a few minutes, depending on how the third stage is managed. There are two approaches to this third stage of labour: physiological and managed.

In a physiological third stage, the focus is on allowing the placenta to separate from the uterine wall and be expelled naturally, without medical intervention. This process usually happens within an hour but can sometimes take longer. Oxytocin plays a key role in contracting the uterus to expel the placenta. In a physiological approach, the body's own production of oxytocin is relied upon to get these contractions started.

If the placenta is taking a while to come away on its own, your midwife may suggest you change to a different position (i.e. sitting on the toilet), or encourage breastfeeding the baby, as it can help to stimulate contractions by promoting the release of more oxytocin. Physiological third stages are preferred in low-risk pregnancies and births, where both mother and baby are stable.

If the placenta is taking longer than expected to come away from the uterus, the midwife will suggest active management in which synthetic oxytocin is used. In a managed third stage, an injection is given into the thigh as soon as the baby is born. It can be given any time after the shoulders are out. The injection usually contains a mixture of syntocinon (the synthetic oxytocin) and ergometrine, a drug used to treat and prevent postpartum haemorrhage. The combined drug is called Syntometrine. In some cases, just syntocinon is used as a single injection.

After the injection is given, the placenta is usually out within 10 minutes. The midwife may apply pressure, called controlled cord traction (CCT), to help guide the placenta out. They will place one hand on your belly to support the uterus, and guide the placenta out with the umbilical cord. This is only successful if the placenta has detached.

Syntometrine is effective at preventing primary postpartum haemorrhage, but does come with side effects such as nausea, headaches, high blood pressure and a higher incidence of readmission for bleeding. Syntometrine is not usually used in cases where someone already has high blood pressure, or they have severe heart, liver or kidney disease. In these cases, syntocinon may be used instead.

A managed third stage may be recommended for some pregnancies where the risk of postpartum haemorrhage is high – for example, those with placenta accreta (a condition where the placenta grows too deep into the uterine wall). If you are unsure which route is best for you, discuss it with your midwife.

Sometimes the placenta doesn't detach properly from the wall of the uterus, regardless of whether the mother has had a physiological or managed third stage. This is called a retained placenta.

A retained placenta needs to be removed in theatre once all other efforts to encourage it to come out of its own accord have been exhausted. This is referred to as a manual removal of the placenta and is done with an epidural or spinal block in place where possible. (A spinal block is one injection of analgesia into the lower spine, commonly given when someone hasn't had an epidural in place throughout their labour.) It occurs in around 1 to 3 per cent of births in the UK and is more common in preterm births.

In most cases, the third stage of labour is relatively uneventful. The placenta coming away can be painful for some but is much less intense than the baby being born. Once detached from the uterus, it is generally expelled easily. The midwife will check to make sure it's complete and there is nothing left inside. They will then check to ensure your uterus is contracted down, and that there is no severe bleeding. At this point, the midwife will also evaluate you for perineal trauma (see page 196).

OPTIMAL CORD CLAMPING

After birth, the baby's umbilical cord is clamped and cut, separating the baby from the placenta. Historically this was done almost instantly, but there is now evidence that babies benefit from a delay before the cord is clamped, allowing at least one minute for extra blood to flow from the placenta into the baby. This is called optimal (or delayed/deferred) cord clamping (OCC) and is beneficial to almost all babies. Although most sources, including the World Health Organization (WHO),[41] recommend one minute, it is ideal to wait several more minutes before clamping to allow the blood to continue flowing through the umbilical vein and for the cord to stop pulsating.

The extra blood from the placenta results in an increased amount of iron being transferred to the baby. Iron is essential for brain development and studies have shown that infants with higher iron levels seem to do better on tests of neurodevelopment later in childhood.[42] The extra blood can also help with a baby's stability after birth.

When the cord is clamped immediately, there is a sudden drop in blood pressure due to the movement of blood into the lungs when the baby takes their first breaths. OCC allows extra blood from the placenta to replace that blood, keeping the pressure more stable. If a caesarean is carried out, delaying cord clamping is possible as long as the baby doesn't need immediate resuscitation.

Amazingly, premature babies benefit even more from OCC. They have more fragile organs, which can be affected by low blood pressure, so improving blood pressure from OCC can help protect these delicate organs and reduce the risk of some of the complications linked to prematurity. Sick babies can also have problems with low blood pressure, so benefit from OCC, too.

There is a small increased risk of jaundice in babies who have received OCC, but this is usually mild and is easily treated by placing the baby under blue light (phototherapy), along with plenty of feeding.

OCC may not be possible to perform if there is an immediate problem with either the mother or baby at the time of birth. In that case, cord clamping will be done straight away so medical treatment can start as soon as possible. If a baby needs a little help after the birth to regulate their breathing or heart rate, the Resuscitation Council recommend attempting to do this with the cord intact on a bed where possible and if safe to do so. This will help the baby by ensuring they are still receiving some oxygen via the placenta.

VERNIX

Vernix caseosa is the white, creamy coating that basically protects the baby's delicate skin from damage that could be caused by prolonged exposure to amniotic fluid. It also has some benefits after the birth, such as keeping the skin supple and hydrated, and potentially helping to protect the baby from infection, so it's a good thing to leave the vernix on the baby. In fact, you can wait for up to two or three days to give the baby their first bath so that the vernix is absorbed naturally into the skin. I know it may seem weird, but you'll have a clean baby really soon. Chester was absolutely covered in vernix but we left it on him, and he had lovely smooth skin.

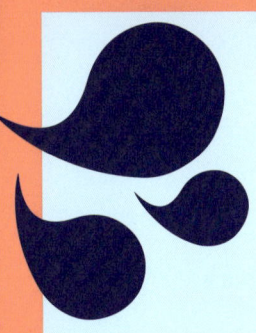

BIRTHING POOLS
AND WATER BIRTHS

I chose to have a birthing pool with all three of my births, and the reason I wanted to use one was because it helps you feel really relaxed. And when you feel relaxed, more pain-relief hormones and fewer stress hormones are triggered – and, as we know, stress and fear are the enemies of labour. The warmth and buoyancy of the water act like natural pain relief. And you can get into some really good positions for labour – you can kneel on the floor of the pool or lean on the side; you can sit down and put your back against the edge of the pool with your arms over the side. Also, studies have shown that because you're in such a relaxed state, the second stage of labour may be shorter and there may be less need for pain medication, so you can be really present.[43] That said, you can use gas and air in the pool if you feel you need it, but you will not be able to have an epidural or use opiates. It's also believed that the water may encourage your body to produce more oxytocin, which helps your rushes work more effectively.

We set up our pool at around 36 weeks just so that it was ready, and actually, it's really exciting looking into a room and seeing the birthing pool there; I spent days just sitting staring at it, imagining myself inside. With Holly, it took me so long to get into active labour that when I did, I was exhausted. I got

into the water when I was 6 or 7cm dilated, but because I was so tired I kept falling asleep in between contractions, just leaning on the pool. And that meant that my labour slowed so I had to get out of the pool to speed it up again, which was heartbreaking as it had felt so warm and soothing in there. With Tilly, I loved being in the pool, and it did provide me with very welcome pain relief.

I found the whole experience of a water birth absolutely joyous. And at one point, the midwife told me to touch between my legs, and I could feel Tilly's hair on her head, just literally crowning, waiting for the next contraction. It gave me the courage and the strength to carry on. I was a little bit worried about what was going to happen to the baby's head when it came out and whether the baby would be able to breathe, but babies continue to get oxygen via the umbilical cord for a few minutes, so they won't try to breathe until you pull them up to the surface, as they think they're still in the amniotic fluid. Once Tilly's head had appeared, I remember Pam saying to me, 'Don't touch the head.' You're advised not to touch it once it's been delivered because if the baby opens their eyes or mouth at this point before their body has arrived, that is when they're at greater risk of waking up and trying to breathe. What's beautiful is that, as I was on my knees, she came out and Pam just pushed her back through my legs up through the front. And I picked her up and sat back in the pool and thought, *Wow, I've done it*. It does feel absolutely miraculous. It's such a beautiful thing for your baby just to rise up through the water into your arms.

The midwife will offer to monitor you and your baby as they would with any other type of birth. They'll have waterproof equipment to monitor the baby's heartbeat, and they'll put a little mirror on the floor of the pool in between your legs to check the baby as it emerges, and see what position its head is in. You can see the mirror, too, and watch the little hairy crown just about to come out, which is so blooming amazing. They'll also check your temperature and the pool's regularly, to make sure you're comfortable and that the pool isn't getting too hot (it shouldn't go above 37.5°C).

Birthing pools come in all shapes and sizes. You can hire them or buy them, and if you hire them, usually they will come with everything you need. There are hiring companies that will cover all things birth – for example, Birth Supplies (homebirthsupplies.co.uk). They will have birthing balls, stools, water-birth accessories, birthing-pool liners – everything you might need.

It's a very personal choice, whether or not to use a birthing pool. Some women would not like to be in water at all or feel safe, but some women who like water (I am a total water baby and love the water) will find it immensely comforting.

'I had the most incredible water birth.' — Lucy

Being in the water was such soothing pain relief. I had some gas and air and worked with my body and baby. Feeling the crown of her head and my husband catching and lifting her from the water was an experience I will never forget.

Davina: I felt exactly the same, Lucy, and I'm so glad it was soothing and calming for you, too. Touching the crown and knowing you're just about to meet your baby is a feeling I wish I could bottle.

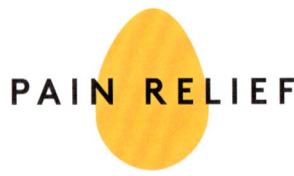

PAIN RELIEF

Okay, let's talk about pain. It's one of the biggies when it comes to birth – every woman wants to know how much it's going to hurt and what they can do about it.

Every single woman's perception of a successful birth looks different but personally I felt like the feeling at the end of giving birth naturally would be so amazing that it would outweigh the pain I would feel without relief, and I wanted that end feeling more than I wanted pain relief. But I do understand that for many women, their idea of a good birth is one where they don't feel the pain. They feel more in control. They are not as scared, and that's why I wanted this book to be completely non-judgmental. You have whatever birth you want to have, because if you're happy, your baby's happy.

When it comes to pain relief, there are lots of different kinds – medical and more natural – and talking through the options with your midwife is going to help you work out what's right for you.

Personally, I was clean from drink and drugs, and I knew there was no way I could take pethidine (which is sometimes used for pain relief in labour) as it's an opioid. I also knew that I didn't want to take gas and air as that is also mood-altering, and I didn't particularly want to have an epidural because I wanted to feel what was happening in my body. But, interestingly, during all three of my labours, just as I was transitioning and about to start pushing, I'd say to my midwife, 'This is when I would ask you for an epidural.' (Even though I was at home and so wouldn't have been able to have one anyway.) And Pam always looked at me and said, 'This is when I would tell you, you don't need one.' And that is because she knew my birth plan. She knew that I just needed a little bit of encouragement to be strong enough not to have the epidural because I didn't really want it. That is what's so amazing about midwives; they know that you would like to go down a certain route and they will encourage you to do just that.

For all of my births, I used a TENS machine (see page 188), which are available to hire, and while I know that, as Marley says, they're not much help in established labour, in the early stage mine definitely helped me because whenever I had a contraction without the TENS machine, it felt noticeably more intense.

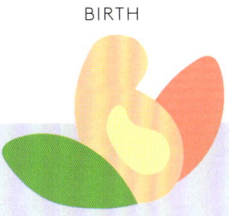

PAIN MANAGEMENT

Midwife Marley

Managing pain during labour is an individual approach, as we all experience the intensity of labour in different ways. Although labour can undoubtedly be an experience that is difficult to put into words, I always encourage women to view each contraction as one step closer to meeting their baby, and not just something that is negative and painful. And while, of course, there is a positive purpose behind contractions, it doesn't make them any less uncomfortable.

I have already discussed hypnobirthing (see page 118), a technique that I highly recommend, but there are other methods of relieving pain.

Pain management doesn't have to begin in the birth centre or hospital, or when the midwife arrives at your home in the case of home births. There are things you can do at home to help in the early stages of labour, such as making use of soothing warm water by taking a bath, having your birth partner massage you and taking paracetamol (do check this first with your care provider).

Pain management options are split into two types – non-pharmacological and pharmacological. Some options can be used simultaneously, and others cannot.

NON-PHARMACOLOGICAL METHODS

Water immersion

Bathing in warm water can help promote relaxation, ease muscle tension and reduce the perception of pain. The warm water can help promote endorphins and oxytocin, and when you focus on this warmth and relaxation, the pain doesn't feel as bad. Buoyancy in water can also make it easier to change positions and move during labour. Some people like to give birth in water by using a birthing pool (see page 184). Many will use the bath at home for much of their labour before their midwife joins them or before heading into the birth centre or hospital. If you use a bath at home during early labour, ensure the water isn't too hot as this can lead to you feeling faint. The water should be less than 37.5°C.

Massage

Back massage and applying pressure to the sacrum (which is the bony region between the tail bone and the base of the spine) with two hands, also known as counter pressure, can be beneficial in relieving pain during labour, particularly if the contractions are mainly felt in the back. To perform counter pressure on the lower back, your birth partner first needs to identify the sacrum. Then, using the heel of the hands, they can place one hand on either side, just above the top of the buttocks. Firmly and steadily apply pressure, and/or move the area in little circles while maintaining the same level of pressure. This can be done during and/or between contractions if necessary.

TENS machine

TENS stands for transcutaneous electrical nerve stimulation. It's a small device you can use, which has electrodes that stick to your back. You can set the device to deliver a small number of electrical impulses that reach your nerves. It is thought that TENS works by encouraging the body to produce endorphins, the body's natural pain relievers. It also limits pain signals sent to the brain.

TENS machines are very popular for use in the early stages of labour. As it progresses, the device may only help as a distraction. TENS machines can be used in conjunction with pharmacological methods of analgesia, such as Entonox and opioids (see below), but cannot be used in water or in conjunction with epidurals. There are no known risks or side effects of TENS devices.

Sterile water injections

There is some evidence to support the use of sterile water injections to the lower back during labour to help with back pain. These injections are only to be carried out by a health professional, and many have reported them to be effective. The midwife will inject small amounts of sterile water into a few points on the lower back during a contraction.

PHARMACOLOGICAL METHODS

Gas and air (Entonox)

Entonox is mixture of nitrous oxide and oxygen that is inhaled through a mask or mouthpiece during contractions. It provides quick relaxation, which in turn can take the edge off any pain experienced. It doesn't take away the sensations completely. It's self-administered, allowing you to control the dosage based on your needs. It has minimal impact on the baby and is not thought to interfere with labour progression, as it doesn't stay in your system for very long. Some women may experience dizziness, nausea or drowsiness as side effects. Entonox can also make you sound a little strange when you speak, so ensure you have sips of water while you're using it to avoid a dry throat.

Opioids

Opioid medications such as pethidine or diamorphine are administered via injection into the muscle or through an intravenous (IV) line. Opioids can help relieve pain and induce relaxation, allowing women to rest between contractions. Those who use opioids during labour may experience effects similar to those from Entonox.

Opioids can cause drowsiness, nausea and dizziness, and usually an anti-sickness medication is given at the same time to reduce the likelihood of nausea and vomiting. They can also cross the placenta, potentially causing drowsiness or respiratory depression in the baby, especially if administered close to birth. This drowsiness after birth can sometimes affect the baby's ability to suckle effectively during the first breastfeed.

Epidural

This involves drugs administered by an anaesthetist via a small catheter into the epidural space in the lower back. A syringe filled with medication is placed in an electronic pump with the catheter attached at one end, leading to the back. The pump automatically controls the amount of medication being delivered into the body. Sometimes top-ups can be given if necessary. The drugs involved in an epidural include a local anaesthetic, such as bupivacaine, and a narcotic, such as fentanyl. When effective, an epidural usually provides complete pain relief. It works by numbing the spinal nerves, subsequently blocking pain signals to the brain. To achieve a total pain block, large quantities are given, which means that it may be difficult to move around, and often you are unable to move from the bed. As epidurals are invasive procedures, it might cause a dip in blood pressure, so the baby's heart rate will need continuous monitoring on a cardiotocograph (CTG) machine. Your blood pressure will be monitored, and you will be given fluids through an IV drip.

Low-dose or 'mobile' epidurals may be an option, but you will need to discuss this with your maternity unit. A low-dose epidural can provide pain relief while allowing you to move around a little. You may be able to go to the toilet, but if you are unable to pass urine, a urinary catheter will be advised.

Epidurals can provide excellent pain relief and can be particularly helpful if you have had a long labour, but they do come with risks. Some of the side effects include itching, nausea, headaches and shivering. In most cases these are short-lived. Epidurals are associated with a higher incidence of assisted births through forceps (see page 207), ventouse (see page 207) and episiotomies (see page 195). Labour is also likely to be slightly longer, mainly the second stage. If you decide to have an epidural, your midwife and anaesthetist will talk through the risks with you. Please note that all the medications listed above are only to be administered or prescribed by a regulated medical professional.

It may be overwhelming looking at these options, and you may be wondering what is best for you. My advice would be to see how you go. You may be adamant that you want an epidural, but when you go into labour, find that using water and Entonox is working well enough for you. Similarly, you may feel that an epidural is out of the question but feel differently as labour progresses. As long as you are informed about all the options and their risks and benefits, you are able to make an informed decision when in labour. Remember, you can change your mind at any time.

YOUR STORIES

'You can plan and dream of your pregnancy and birth being a certain way, but we are resilient, and some things are out of our control. Be kind to yourself and fight for what you may be able to control while you know your baby is not in harm's way.' — Julianne

It may be overwhelming looking at all these different options, and you may be wondering what is best for you.

My advice would be to see how you go.

As long as you are informed about all the different options, the risks and the benefits, you are able to make an informed decision when in labour.

Remember, you can change your mind at any time.

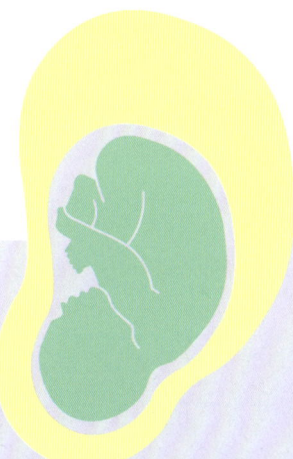

YOUR BABY'S POSITION

Midwife Marley

The most common and optimal position for a baby to be in for birth is head down (cephalic), with the spine facing your belly. This is known as an occiput anterior position. The chin should be tucked into the baby's chest, which makes birthing the head easier.

While the vast majority of babies adopt this position in time for labour, many don't. Alternative positions don't always necessarily mean a vaginal birth is out of the question, but certain positions can make labour longer and trickier.

There are several things the midwife will want to know when caring for you during labour, in relation to how baby is positioned in your womb. They will look at the presentation, lie and overall position of the baby to ensure as smooth a birth as possible.

— **Presentation:** This refers to the part of the baby that is presenting closest to the cervix: if it's the head, it's cephalic; if it's the buttocks, legs or knees, it's breech. On rare occasions, the shoulder can present first.

— **Lie:** The foetal lie refers to the position of the baby inside the mother's womb in relation to the mother's spine. It describes whether the baby is lying longitudinally (vertical), transversely (horizontal) or oblique (diagonally) in the uterus. Ideally, the baby should be lying longitudinally.

— **Position:** This refers to the position of the presenting part of the baby in relation to the pelvis. If the baby is in a head-down, longitudinal position and the crown of the head (occiput) is facing the front of the pelvis, it's referred to as occiput anterior (OA). If the occiput is slightly off to the left, it's called left occiput anterior (LOA). These are both optimal birth positions. If the occiput is facing the back of the pelvis, it is called occiput posterior (OP). You may well hear this being called 'sunny side up' or 'back to back', as the baby's spine is running along the mother's. This position can sometimes make labour longer, and there is a higher change of prodromal labour (see page 170).

If the baby is in a breech position, your obstetric doctor may offer you an external cephalic version (ECV), which is where they manually manipulate the position of the baby during pregnancy with ultrasound guidance. This procedure can be uncomfortable and 1 in 200 babies will need an emergency caesarean immediately after the procedure due to foetal distress.

The other options are either to have a vaginal birth with professionals experienced in managing breech labours, or a planned caesarean.

CAN YOU GET YOUR BODY INTO AN OPTIMAL BIRTHING POSITION?

There are positions you can adopt during pregnancy to help get your baby into an optimal birthing position. When resting, pop a pillow between your knees and lie on your left side.

Try yoga positions such as 'child's pose', and kneel on the floor with your body and arms leaning over the sofa or a bean bag for a few minutes each day. There are also positions you can check out at milescircuit.com, which might be useful.

Moxibustion, a form of reflexology, has also been reported as being useful in turning breech babies; however, there is not enough concrete evidence to support its efficacy.

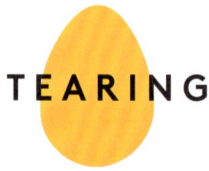

TEARING

Ideally, as I mentioned earlier, if you're having a vaginal birth, you really want to try and help your babies be born slowly and gently. The reason giving birth stings so much is because your skin is having to stretch to make space for the baby's head to come out, so you want to give your vagina and perineum time to do that. But with Holly I had to get her out quite quickly, so I didn't have time, and I did have a small second-degree tear. Marley is going to explain more about tearing, the different degrees and what they mean, but mine meant that I was torn inside and out. And tearing was a big fear for me; I just thought the pain would be so intense. But after Holly had come out, I looked at the midwife and said triumphantly, 'I didn't tear!' What was I afraid of, I didn't even feel it? She looked at me and said, 'You did, but you've done great and don't worry, we can look after you and everything will be fine.' My tear was considered small enough to heal without stitches (Holly weighed 3.68kg/8lb 12oz) and I did manage to heal it by taking it easy. Not by going to the supermarket to show off my new baby, which is what I wanted to do, but by staying in my pyjamas, staying near bed or in bed, and really, really taking it easy for ten days. And what was interesting was that when I went back to see my GP for my check-up at six weeks, they said, 'Wow, those stitches were amazing. They're so neat. Your scar is perfect.' I said, 'I didn't have any stitches. It just healed.' And I'm so grateful for that. The second time, with Tilly (she was 4.39kg/9lb 11oz), I had a first-degree tear, which was just a little bit of a tear around my perineum; I didn't really notice it. And the third time, with Chester (4.59kg/10lb 2oz), I didn't tear at all (I was like a wizard's sleeve, ha ha).

I know there can be a lot of fear around perineal tearing – and while I can't speak for what third- or fourth-degree tears are like, I want to try to reassure you that in my experience the fear of the smaller tears does feel worse than the reality. And if you really allow your body time to heal and rest, they will usually heal after a few weeks.

> ## I looked at the midwife and said, 'I didn't tear!' She looked at me and said, 'You did, but you've done great.'

TYPES OF TEARING

Marley: Around 90 per cent of first-time mums having a vaginal birth will experience some form of trauma to the perineum, labia or vagina. Although this sounds like a relatively scary statistic, the majority of these injuries will be minor tears or grazes that heal quickly. The incidence of tears reduces with subsequent babies.

Perineal tears are far more common than vaginal or labial tears, and are separated into four different categories:

— **First degree:** A minor tear to the skin, similar to a cut on the hand or leg that doesn't need stitches. Most people won't even notice them and they heal relatively quickly.

— **Second degree:** The tear goes into the skin and some of the muscle. These tears will often need some stitches but usually heal well without complications. Suturing is carried out in the same room as the birth, with a local anaesthetic.

— **Third degree:** These tears are deeper, reaching into the anal sphincter. They require suturing in theatre with adequate analgesia, such as an epidural or spinal block.

— **Fourth degree:** These are the least common, with the tear reaching through the anal sphincter, into the rectum. Like third-degree tears, repair in theatre is necessary.

Third- and fourth-degree tears occur in less than 3 per cent of vaginal births and can take many weeks to heal. Both are more likely if you have an assisted birth with forceps or ventouse, if the baby is facing up rather than down (back to back), and if the baby is large – it's important to note, however, that most bigger babies are born without third- and fourth-degree tearing, and I've personally helped a 4.99kg (11lb) baby into the world, which resulted in no tears whatsoever! Physiotherapy postnatally is often needed to help prevent continence issues resulting from third- and fourth-degree tears. If you have a third- or fourth-degree tear, there is a chance of future perineal injury with subsequent births, so any care during future pregnancies is usually discussed with an obstetric doctor to help you plan for the next birth.

EPISIOTOMY

An episiotomy is a cut to the perineum, which is carried out by the midwife or obstetric doctor during the birth of the baby's head. In the UK it's usually only done if there is a need to expedite the birth with the use of instruments such as forceps, or sometimes if the baby's shoulder is stuck and the doctor or midwife need room to perform manoeuvres to free the shoulder. A cut is made at an angle to prevent the wound from tearing further towards the anus. Episiotomies can take longer than spontaneous tears to heal and they can only be carried out with your explicit consent.

There are some things that can be done to help reduce the chance of perineal trauma and the need for an episiotomy:

— Perineal massage during pregnancy (see page 153).

— Using a warm compress during the pushing stage may help with perineal stretching.

— Giving birth kneeling, on all fours or in a side-lying position.

Practising breathing techniques during pregnancy can also help you remain in control during the pushing stage so that you work with your body's pushing reflex to breathe your baby down, allowing for the perineum to slowly stretch during contractions. (For more on breathing techniques, see page 37.)

'My greatest wish was to end my low-risk pregnancy in a birth centre.' — Petra

YOUR STORIES

Unfortunately, due to high blood pressure in the third trimester, I ended up having a hospital birth. Everything turned out completely different than I had imagined. I wanted to move freely – but I was stuck on the CTG. I preferred to tear naturally, but got an episiotomy and forceps. Everything was decided very quickly. Despite all the circumstances, the birth remains positive in my mind. Everyone involved was really nice and relaxed, and after the birth everything went according to my expectations.

Delayed cord clamping, immediate skin to skin, delayed weighing, etc. And we went home on the same day :)

Davina: Petra, it's really interesting hearing somebody who had quite solidly planned out what they wanted, and then everything turned out differently, but you still remained positive. That's so helpful to hear and to try and hold on to the things that you wanted to happen, that did happen and that gave you an overall positive memory. Thanks so much.

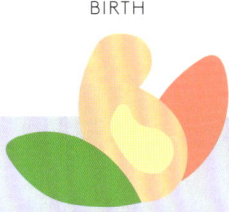

INDUCTION AND AUGMENTATION OF LABOUR

Midwife Marley

An induction is ultimately an intervention that involves starting the labour process through drugs or medical procedures, and augmentation is speeding up the labour process in a person whose labour has stalled or slowed down. This section will help you consider some of the risks and benefits in case you need to make a decision about them.

Inductions are mainly offered for a few reasons:

— There is a medical need. The risk of you remaining pregnant outweighs the risk of you being induced. This could be because of things like ICP (see page 146), or severe pre-eclampsia (see page 144).

— The pregnancy has gone on longer than 41 weeks.

— The baby is expected to be large, in conjunction with other medical issues.

— Pre-labour rupture of membranes (PROM) has occurred, which means that the waters have broken but labour hasn't started and it's been over 24 hours.

All situations are unique and the decision you make regarding induction will be, too. Your doctor and/or midwife will discuss your particular pregnancy with you to identify any potential benefits of induction, along with the risks.

It is very common to be offered an induction when a pregnancy continues after 41 weeks. This is because some research has identified that pregnancies that typically last longer have a slightly increased chance of complications. This does not mean that it is a 'bad' thing to give birth at 42 weeks, or that if you don't go into labour by 40 weeks, something negative will occur. For healthy pregnancies, it is impossible to predict whether it would be beneficial for that particular mother and baby to induce them or wait for labour to start on its own. Pregnancies typically last between 37 and 42 weeks with 80 per cent arriving before the end of the 40th week and 99 per cent arriving before the end of the 41st week. Factors that can affect the time you go into labour include genetics (consider the length of any previous pregnancies or those of your immediate female relatives), height (taller women tend to carry babies for longer) and ethnicity (Black and Asian women may have a shorter overall gestational period than white women).

I always encourage people to ask questions about their specific situation when talking about induction, seeking clarification on the benefits and risks with their healthcare provider, along with any potential alternatives, including waiting for natural labour. This can help you decide if induction for a pregnancy that goes past your due date is something you wish to do.

HOW IS AN INDUCTION OF LABOUR PERFORMED?

This depends very much on what your body is doing on the day of induction; it is always carried out in a hospital setting.

The first step is to make sure you and your baby are well. After an initial wellbeing check of your baby's heart rate and maternal observations, the midwife will perform a vaginal examination to check for any changes to the cervix. If the cervix is long, hard and closed, they will use a prostaglandin gel or pessary to help 'ripen' it. This softens the cervix, encouraging it to shorten and dilate. Some hospitals offer pessaries that are left in the vagina for up to 24 hours and you may be able to go home and await labour. Do check with the hospital to see if this is something they offer.

Prostaglandin pessaries aren't the only way to 'ripen' and dilate the cervix; mechanical options such as dilapan rods and foley balloons are alternatives. These are devices that are placed in the cervix to slowly dilate it over a period of time. Your healthcare provider will discuss all of the options and process with you, before commencing an induction.

Labour may begin from this alone with nothing else required. Alternatively, it may help with opening the cervix but fall short of starting any contractions. If this is the case, the next step would be to break the waters with a thin plastic tool that is passed through the cervix to nick the membrane sac. If the contractions still do not begin after this stage, a synthetic oxytocin drip called syntocinon is given intravenously via your arm. This quickly causes the uterus to start contracting and the dose is increased periodically until contractions are coming every three minutes. Oxytocin is the hormone that is produced naturally by the brain and increases drastically during labour, stimulating contractions. Synthetic oxytocin is a drug that mimics oxytocin (see page 169).

If the cervix has already started to dilate when you initially attend the hospital to begin your induction, prostaglandins aren't usually necessary. The midwife will use something called a Bishop score[44] to assess the cervix and identify whether the pessary is needed. If not, they will skip that stage and go straight to breaking the bag. If you have arrived after your waters have broken for the labour to be augmented as 24 hours have passed, they will go straight to setting up the synthetic oxytocin drip.

Induction of labour is not necessarily a quick process. It can sometimes go on for several days, particularly if the body is not ready. Occasionally the prostaglandins don't work to change the cervix at all. The membranes cannot be ruptured, and the synthetic oxytocin cannot be administered until the cervix has started to change. If this happens, the next course of action will be discussed with you by your obstetric doctor.

Synthetic oxytocin can cause powerful contractions. While some women cope with them, many will need strong forms of analgesia, such as epidural (see page 189). While on the oxytocin drip, the baby will need to be monitored continuously to make sure it is coping with the contractions, and that you are not having too many in a short space of time. There is also a small risk of uterine rupture, but your midwife will be with you at all times to monitor you and your baby.

Labour augmentation uses the same techniques as labour induction but is offered for different reasons. When a labour has already begun, but has slowed down or stalled, the midwife or doctor may suggest breaking your waters or putting the syntocinon drip up to encourage regular contractions. Before I talk more about augmenting labour, it's good to remember that the length of labour will be different in everyone. Some people will have an established labour that lasts two hours, while for others it may last 10 hours or more. There is a guideline used in hospitals for labour progress that midwives and doctors use, called a partogram. This chart keeps an eye on things like the number, strength and length of contractions, the baby's heart activity, and the mother's heart rate, blood pressure, respiratory rate and temperature, cervical dilation and overall wellbeing. It helps midwives and doctors recognise unusual patterns during labour that might need attention or intervention.

There are a number of reasons why labour may progress slowly or stall, but often it's because of the positioning of the baby. Foetal position will be discussed further in another section (see page 192), but ultimately, if the crown of the head (occiput) isn't aligned well with the cervix to be able to put enough pressure on it, or the head is too high and struggling to come down lower into the birth canal, the uterus may struggle to contract effectively. Fear and tension may also inhibit the release of natural oxytocin, required for the uterus to contract. Before jumping straight into administering drugs for augmentation or rupturing the membranes, your midwife may discuss changes of position to see if that creates more space for the baby to get into an optimal position. Oxytocin release is also encouraged through nipple stimulation, so it is not uncommon for midwives to suggest using a breast pump or rolling the nipples between your fingers to increase contractions.

If a labour is moving slowly but there are no concerns with the mum or baby, a change of position, rest and hydration may be enough to get things kickstarted again.

YOUR STORIES

'I had IVF to have my first born. I really wanted to have a natural birth but ended up with a C-section as I only got to 2cm dilation.' — Vicky

The consultant was insistent on me being induced when my dating scan suggested I was overdue rather than when my IVF predicted date was. Despite doing everything to avoid induction, I ended up having one, which was the start of

a birthing journey I was desperate to avoid. I needed medical intervention throughout. I was stressed and anxious. Despite the C-section going well, I ended up having an internal bleed that left me quite traumatised and unwell. I wasn't offered a debrief and now, with my second IVF baby due, I feel the same anxiety returning as I get closer to my due date. What I have learned is that women need to feel empowered in their journey, as it's their most vulnerable time. Consultants must listen and work out a plan together with mothers.

Davina: Vicky, thanks so much for talking about this. I would imagine that after a first traumatic birth, the second one is a real worry, and women need to do a lot of thinking and planning on how to make the next birth, if you have one, a calmer and more pleasant one for you.

YOUR STORIES

'I was 10 days overdue when my waters broke. I went in but wasn't in labour so was sent home and was told that if I was not having contractions within 24 hours to return.' — Louise

I lasted at home as long as I could by taking a warm bath; eventually I went back in and was only 4 to 5cm dilated. Fast forward another one and a half hours and there was still no progress so I was informed I would need a C-section. I was very upset at this as it wasn't how I imagined my birth, as the baby was in no immediate distress. They let me wait another hour, which I am most grateful for as I think they knew the end outcome would be the same, but they allowed me that time to process and realise it was the best thing. The procedure was pain-free and when I was shown my 4.5kg (10lb) (!!) baby I was instantly in love and grateful he hadn't come vaginally. I felt looked after and supported post op and my birth experience, while not what I had in mind, was extremely positive. So much so I elected for a C-section with the next one!'

Davina: Thank you for sharing your story, Louise. I think it's really valuable to hear about when a labour doesn't end up progressing as you had hoped it would or planned, but that that isn't necessarily a bad thing. To know that you were pleased you ended up having a C-section is a good outcome to a sensitive and troubling time. I'm so glad that you had a positive ending to your story.

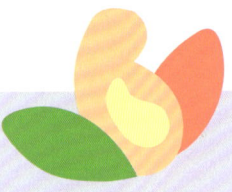

MEMBRANE SWEEPS

Midwife Marley

Membrane sweeps, also referred to as stripping the membranes, is a procedure that is sometimes offered at full term if your pregnancy goes past your 'due date', as a way to encourage the body to go into labour, avoiding a medical induction. Membrane sweeps are a form of labour induction, just without drugs. The midwife or doctor will use two fingers inserted into the vagina to reach through the cervix so that they can feel the membrane sac around the baby's head. They will then move their fingers in a circular or 'sweeping' motion, separating the membranes from the base of the cervix. This is thought to stimulate the production of prostaglandins, a hormone released by the cervix that encourages softening and dilation. A membrane sweep can only be achieved if the cervix has already started to open. For many women, first-time mums in particular, the cervix remains closed until the start of labour, meaning a membrane sweep cannot be performed.

The discussion around membrane sweeps usually begins at around week 38 to 39 in your pregnancy, along with medical induction of labour. Although they are commonly performed at around 40 weeks if there is no sign of labour, they are more effective when performed after 41 weeks of pregnancy, with around 50 per cent of women going into labour within 48 hours of having one at that stage.

Membrane sweeps are offered to everyone, but you can choose to wait for labour to start naturally if you prefer. Some people will be offered a membrane sweep earlier than their due date if there are factors that indicate that an induction of labour is recommended early, such as pre-eclampsia (see page 144).

A membrane sweep can be repeated at intervals of several days if not effective. As with any invasive procedure, membrane sweeps do come with small risks, including discomfort, light bleeding, irregular contractions that may not lead to labour and, as with all vaginal examinations, infection.

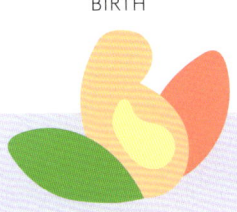

MONITORING IN LABOUR

Midwife Marley

During labour, the midwife will be keeping an eye on the wellbeing of the baby by offering to monitor the heart rate. They will also ask you to keep an eye on the baby's movements, although you may struggle to notice much when you are having contractions! It's not only the baby that we need to keep an eye on – the midwife will be assessing your wellbeing by taking your blood pressure and temperature, making sure you're passing urine regularly, and making note of any vaginal losses like blood or amniotic fluid.

There are several ways in which the midwife can monitor the baby's heart rate. A hand-held electrical Doppler or Pinard stethoscope allows the midwife to listen in via the outside of the abdomen, every 15 minutes in established labour, so that the heart rate can be documented in relation to the contractions. The probe of the Doppler or Pinard is held against the belly at the point where the midwife thinks the baby's chest might be. The midwife will listen for around 60 seconds after a contraction. To ensure the midwife has definitely picked up the heart rate of the baby, they will measure your pulse at the same time. If any unusual heartbeats are detected, they may ask you to change into a different position or encourage you to drink water. Sometimes these things help to resolve minor changes in the heart rate.

If persistent abnormal heart sounds are heard, a cardiotocograph (CTG) monitor may be suggested, as this offers a consistent trace of the baby's heart rate. A CTG is a device that is placed on your abdomen to collect information about the baby's heart rate and your contractions. It isn't used if the labour is straightforward and there are no concerns. Aside from using it when there are concerns after using a hand-held Doppler or Pinard stethoscope, it may be used in the following scenarios (this list is not exhaustive):

— Induction of labour

— Epidural

— Pregnancy with multiples

— Bleeding during labour

— Women with diabetes who are on IV medication through labour

— Those who have had previous caesareans

— Babies who are growth-restricted

There are other indications for CTG monitoring, and your midwife will discuss this with you if the situation arises.

Sometimes it is difficult to hear the heart rate effectively outside of the body with the external transducers. If it's difficult to pick up and a CTG has been recommended, a foetal scalp electrode may be indicated. This device has a metal spiral wire on the end that attaches to the baby's head via the cervix. The foetal scalp electrode collects information about the baby's heart rate, which is recorded on the CTG machine.

CTG machines are usually wired, meaning movement during labour is often limited. Limiting your movement can be uncomfortable when your body is telling you to get into a particular position, so if you are on a wired CTG, your midwife may suggest sitting on a birthing ball close to the machine or kneeling on the bed. You may also be able to stand up, enabling you to rock your hips from side to side, which some women find useful during contractions.

Some maternity units use wireless devices for CTG, which means that full movement is possible as there are no wires restricting you.

It is very important to know that vaginal examinations are not obligatory. In fact, no examination, intervention, medication or investigation can be performed without your full consent.

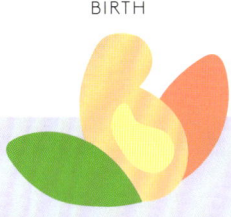

VAGINAL EXAMINATIONS DURING LABOUR

Midwife Marley

Vaginal examinations (VE) are routinely offered at the start of and throughout labour to evaluate the cervix. During a VE, a midwife or doctor places two fingers inside the vagina to check the dilation, effacement (or thinning) and position of the cervix, the position of the presenting part (usually the head) and the station of the baby's head in relation to the pelvis. This gives them an idea of how labour is progressing, in conjunction with other things like contractions.

When it is thought that you could be in labour, VEs are frequently carried out as part of the initial labour assessment. Guidance states that VEs should be offered every four hours once labour has been established, unless otherwise indicated.

It is very important to know that vaginal examinations are not obligatory. In fact, no examination, intervention, medication or investigation can be performed without your full consent.

Although vaginal examinations can be useful for the midwife or doctor in assessing progress, they are often not essential in straightforward labours. There are, however, scenarios where an intervention cannot be carried out without a vaginal examination first – for example, induction of labour (see page 197).

Vaginal examinations can sometimes be uncomfortable and pose a small risk of membrane rupture and infection. If you have concerns around vaginal examinations, discuss these with your midwife prior to labour when going through your birth plan.

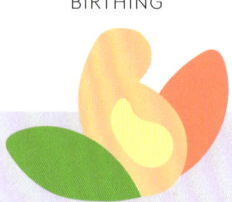

COMPLICATIONS AND ASSISTED BIRTHS

Midwife Marley

Sometimes, labour doesn't run as smoothly as hoped and there may be a need for interventions. Some examples of potential complications include:

Placental abruption: The placenta begins to detach from the uterus, affecting the baby's heart rate. There may be bleeding present but not always. Depending on the stage of labour and the wellbeing of the mum and baby, a caesarean may be indicated. Placental abruption occurs in approximately 1 per cent of pregnancies, usually in the third trimester.

Uterine abruption: This is extremely rare, occurring in around 1 in 5,000 pregnancies. The uterus forms a small tear. This is more likely to occur in people who have had their labour induced, and those who have had previous caesareans or uterine surgery. An urgent caesarean is usually performed in these cases.

Obstructed labour: If the labour is unusually long, it could be because of an obstruction. This is a situation where the baby is unable to descend into the pelvis properly, despite strong, regular contractions. The most common cause is misalignment of the presenting part of the baby. The head may be extended with the chin up and head tilted back, tilted to the side, or perhaps the baby is lying in a transverse position so is unable to enter the pelvis. Many hospitals are now adopting birth biomechanics, encouraging birthing women to move around and get into different positions to help the baby align properly with the pelvis if a slight obstruction is suspected.

Rarely, the baby's head is too large to fit through the pelvis. This is called cephalo-pelvic disproportion (CPD). This term has historically been overused and many women have undergone caesareans unnecessarily with a false diagnosis of CPD. The true incidence of CPD is unclear, but it's thought to be less than 0.001 per cent.

Foetal distress: This term is used during pregnancy or labour to describe warning signs that the baby might be unwell. In labour this could be abnormalities with the heart rate. Some fluctuations in the heart rate are expected, particularly with contractions and during the pushing stage. Some minor fluctuations with the heart rate occur because the baby has been lying on the umbilical cord, or if you are dehydrated, and are resolved with a change of position and by drinking water or administering IV fluids. If the midwife or doctor suspects there is an underlying issue, they may suggest doing further tests, which involve checking the baby's blood oxygen levels. If it's thought that the baby isn't getting enough oxygen, an urgent birth will be recommended. This is usually in the form of an emergency caesarean if the person is still in the first stage of labour, or an assisted birth with forceps or ventouse (see below) if pushing in the second stage has already begun.

Shoulder dystocia: This occurs when the baby's shoulder gets stuck on the brim of the pelvis, preventing the body being born. If the midwife suspects shoulder dystocia, they will likely ask you to bring your knees to your chest to help release the shoulder. There are other manoeuvres, such as turning you onto all fours and applying pressure just above your pubic bone, that can help.

Assisted births are methods used to help with the birth of a baby when labour isn't progressing smoothly or there's a need to expedite the process. These interventions are typically performed by obstetric doctors. There are two methods used:

— **Forceps** are specialised instruments resembling large spoons or tongs. They're carefully applied to the baby's head inside the vagina to help guide the baby out during contractions. Forceps are likely to leave a temporary mark or bruise on the baby's face. You are also likely to need an episiotomy with forceps.

— **Ventouse**, also known as vacuum extraction, involves using a vacuum cup attached to a suction device. The cup is placed on the baby's head, and suction is applied to help grip the head securely. As the mother pushes during contractions, the healthcare provider gently pulls on the ventouse to assist in bringing the baby out. Babies who are born via vacuum will usually have a temporary swelling on the head, which resolves within 24 hours. They are also more likely to develop jaundice.

Babies born via an assisted birth may find feeding difficult in the early days. This might be due to discomfort on their heads due to the forceps or suction devices. Support should be offered to you, particularly if you are breastfeeding – a paediatric doctor should assess the pain and provide relief and a lactation consultant should assist with breastfeeding.

When a complication or emergency arises, the midwife may press the buzzer on the wall of the birthing room. This can be overwhelming as the room quickly becomes full of health professionals who arrive to assist. If you are at home and a complication arises, most of the time the midwife can pre-empt it and will call an ambulance for a transfer to hospital. They will also call the maternity unit so that they are waiting when you arrive. Home-birth midwives are trained for emergency situations.

On rare occasions, emergencies arise without warning. Some, however, are as a result of interventions carried out in hospital, such as induction of labour (see page 197). This is why it is important to understand both the benefits and risks of all interventions offered, helping you to make an informed choice. Health professionals will know the risks involved with interventions and will monitor you accordingly.

YOUR STORIES

'I did hypnobirthing, which was amazing and really got me through.' — Abby

However, I was advised to be induced due to a big baby. Unfortunately, this made my labour really long and painful. I eventually got to the birthing suite, but my baby's head was sideways. They discovered this after two hours of pushing. I had to go to theatre so they could try forceps and suction, but this didn't work. I ended up with an emergency C-section. After really enjoying my pregnancy and learning about hypnobirthing, I unfortunately ended up with a birth I didn't want, which was also quite traumatic. Also, the baby wasn't even *big – in the end he was 7lb 5oz! I really wish I had stayed strong and said no to an induction. This was my first baby, so I went with the medical advice.*

Davina: Abby's story is such a powerful reminder of how important it is that we advocate for ourselves – and have the courage to stand up for what we want and what we feel is right. Abby, I really hope your experience will help other women to fight for the interventions they do and don't want.

PEOPLE PLEASING AND VOICING YOUR WISHES

I want to talk a little bit about speaking up because if, like me, you are a bit of a people pleaser, you will find it very hard to say no or ask for what you want or need. And when you are giving birth, it is really important that you do feel able and empowered to vocalise exactly what you need at each moment.

If you recognise yourself in any of the behaviours below, you might be a people pleaser:

You have a difficult time saying no

You worry what other people might think

You feel guilty saying no to people

You think that saying no will make people think that you're selfish

You agree to things you don't like or don't want to do

You have feelings of low self-esteem

You say sorry all the time

You don't have much free time because you're always doing things for other people

You neglect your own needs and desires in order to do things for others

If you feel that you are not being listened to, you can ask to speak to a different member of staff. Helping yourself feel empowered and safe/secure will be guided by how you speak, so just talking calmly and clearly can go a long way towards making sure you're being heard and listened to.

Do not accept having somebody at your labour because they are insisting on it. Often in-laws are very keen to be at labours and they think they're helping, but if you don't want them there, don't let them come. You might need to ask your partner for some help with that.

'For my first pregnancy, I really wanted to have a caesarean. I'm not sure why but I think fears around being a Black woman accessing services can be scary, so I think I felt in more control.' — Simphiwe

Friends and family thought I was being ridiculous because I was young, so in the end I opted for a natural birth but unfortunately during labour things escalated and I had to have an emergency caesarean and both baby and I had sepsis, so a poorly start to our journey.

With my second child I had a planned caesarean, but through my pregnancy we needed a lot of support from the trauma team as both my husband and I were very worried about the birth. I do feel that the team was mindful of our previous birth and when I reported concerns, they were generally listened to. I think being in labour on Christmas Day was scary as working within the NHS I know there is a skeleton staff during the festive season. But we had our planned caesarean. It was like a spa day: we had the music of our choice, walked to theatre; it was much calmer than being rushed and bells are being rung and people are running and rushing around. It wasn't perfect but I'm grateful to be alive and to hold my baby at the end of it all.

Davina: Simphiwe, thank you so much for all the work that you do. It's been so nice getting to know you as a friend and a colleague, but I also really want to thank you for sharing your story with us.

I wholeheartedly believe that elective caesareans are a brilliant way forward when you've experienced a very traumatic birth, and I love your description of your second elective caesarean and how it was like a spa day.

I'm really pleased to have a story like this in the book, because you work in the medical field, and I hope your words will be really reassuring for others. Big hugs.

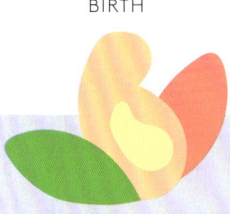

CAESAREAN BIRTH (PLANNED AND UNPLANNED)

Midwife Marley

Some women will give birth abdominally, via caesarean, also known as C-section. A caesarean is a surgical procedure carried out in an operating theatre that involves cutting through the lower abdomen to reach the baby. They are commonly carried out under regional anaesthesia in the back, such as an epidural or spinal block. In some situations, a general anaesthetic is used to put you to sleep. This may be the case when there is no time to wait for a spinal, or if there are reasons why one cannot be given (for example, in the incidence of some blood-clotting disorders).

Caesareans are either carried out as planned (elective) or unplanned (emergency):

— **Planned:** Reasons for a planned caesarean include a maternal request due to fear of birth, previous birth trauma or a previous caesarean, breech or transverse lie (see page 206), placenta praevia (see page 147), or another factor that may raise safety concerns over a vaginal birth, such as some maternal heart conditions.

— **Unplanned:** Reasons include (in addition to some of the emergency situations previously mentioned) active maternal herpes to prevent transmission to the baby, preterm pregnancies or growth restriction where an urgent birth is required but induction is too risky, and some cases of severe pre-eclampsia (see page 144).

If you are faced with making a decision on an unplanned caesarean unexpectedly, it may feel disappointing if it doesn't align with the birth experience you were hoping for. Please rest assured, there is often nothing that you could have done differently. If you feel this way, speaking to someone for a birth debrief might be helpful, and there is more information on this on page 224. When writing a birth plan (see page 100), you can include your wishes in unforeseen circumstances.

This may help you when it comes to managing your expectations.

If you are planning on having a caesarean, your maternity team may ask you to prepare beforehand by:

— not eating for several hours prior to hospital admission

— shaving the area by your pubic bone, although some hospitals may ask you to wait for it to be done on the day

— making sure you leave all jewellery at home and remove any nail varnish.

They may also provide you with anti-reflux medication to take on the morning of your surgery. You will have a pre-op assessment, when the medical team will go through a consent form and there will be a review by an anaesthetist. Blood tests are also usually carried out prior to surgery.

If the caesarean is unplanned, you will still need to consent to it verbally and in writing. The only time verbal and written consent isn't required is if you are unconscious and do not have capacity to do so.

During the surgery, you are taken into theatre by the midwife and will be greeted by a team of people, including an anaesthetist, operating department practitioner (ODP), the surgeon (obstetric doctor) and their assistant, who is another doctor, and an assistant who may be a healthcare assistant or maternity support worker. If there are concerns for the baby, a neonatal paediatric doctor may also be called in.

The anaesthetist is there to make sure you are numb from the waist down and that all of your vital signs are okay throughout the operation. If you already have an epidural in place from being in labour, they will top it up so that you are completely numb. If not, they will administer a spinal block, which is an injection into the lower back with the same effect as an epidural. During this time, your birth partner will likely be getting changed into scrubs, ready to come into theatre and join you. If you require a general anaesthetic, most hospitals do not permit birth partners in theatre. If the baby is well, they will usually bring them out to the birth partner in recovery, to wait until the mum wakes up.

The actual procedure of getting the baby and placenta out of the womb takes less than 10 minutes in straightforward caesareans. You will be in theatre for up to an hour as they complete the suturing. During this time, you will still feel numb but should be able to hold the baby with support from your birth partner and midwife. Skin-to-skin contact with the baby should be possible if there are no concerns, and your midwife will be able to help with this. After surgery, you are taken into recovery, where you will stay for a while before being taken to the main postnatal ward. In recovery you will get support with feeding your baby, and your midwife will advise when it's okay for you to eat and drink.

Post-caesarean itching and shakiness are common as a result of the spinal/epidural medications. Your stay in hospital may be anywhere between one and two days for a straightforward caesarean, or longer if there are complications (see page 224). If your baby requires a long stay in the NICU, you will be discharged from hospital when well enough, and will be able to visit your baby at any time.

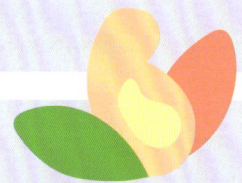

VAGINAL BIRTH AFTER CAESAREAN (VBAC)

Midwife Marley

After having a caesarean, you may wonder if it's possible to have a vaginal birth with your next pregnancy. The answer is yes, it is, and it is called a vaginal birth after caesarean (VBAC). Studies have shown a 60 to 80 per cent success rate for VBAC, which is a positive sign for women hoping to give birth vaginally during their next birth. There are pre-existing factors, which will add to the chance of success.

These include:

— having at least 18 months between the C-section and next birth

— having had a vaginal birth before your C-section (you can still have a VBAC if you haven't)

— not having any special circumstances in the pregnancy, such as placenta praevia (see page 147), fibroids, breech baby at full term or twins on board

— having a BMI of 18 to 30

In subsequent pregnancies where a VBAC is desired, the hospital will refer you to a 'VBAC clinic' or 'VBAC talk' where all the facts about having a vaginal birth after caesarean are discussed. This will help with the decision-making process. The main concern about VBAC is the 0.5 per cent risk of uterine rupture. This does mean, however, that you will have a 99.5 per cent chance of not having a uterine rupture. The main difference with someone in labour attempting a VBAC is that there will be continuous foetal monitoring. This can help to identify any potential problems that may occur.

A VBAC is not recommended for people who had a classical incision during their caesarean (a vertical cut as opposed to horizontal), or if they've previously had a uterine rupture or uterine surgery, such as fibroid removal.

YOUR STORIES

'This was my fourth pregnancy but the first to make it this far.' — Demi

Being pregnant after baby loss was a challenging thing to navigate. Every day I was scared this baby was going to die, too. I felt I had lost all confidence in my body and was desperate to bring a baby home. I chose an elective, gentle C-section and it was amazing. I remember walking into theatre and having to sit down because I was so overwhelmed. What a strange thing

214

to have someone cut through seven layers while you're awake. Women and birthing people are so incredible. If you're wondering what a gentle C-section entails, then I'll explain how mine went. I had the drapes dropped so I could watch my daughter enter the world. She came out slowly and gently and received delayed cord clamping; the process from where her head was out to the moment she was in my arms was approximately 10 minutes. The surgeons were so respectful of my wishes, and I felt calm throughout. It was a really empowering experience after so much heartache.

Hearing my baby cry felt surreal. I couldn't believe it. The birth of my daughter changed my life forever. I was calm, in control, and the moment she was placed onto my chest I felt peace.

Davina: Thanks for your story, Demi. This was the first time I'd heard about an elective, gentle C-section, and it sounds absolutely lovely. And I'm so pleased that you felt empowered after everything that you'd been through. Lots of love.

YOUR STORIES

'Four months ago I had a gentle C-section (elective) after a difficult pregnancy with many complications and nine months of stress and dread.' — Michelle

The experience of the C-section was beyond amazing! I loved every moment of it as I got to watch my son be born. Seeing him gently make his way out of my womb as my husband and I watched was surreal and magical. The theatre team were unbelievable and made me feel so safe, seen and heard. My midwife on the day was only 21 years old but she filled us with confidence and made the whole experience enjoyable (believe it or not).

Davina: Michelle, it's so important to tell positive C-section stories because for so many women this is a fantastic way to give birth and is what suits their situation best. I'm so pleased your experience was brilliant, and I love that you highlighted that it doesn't matter how old a midwife is. They can still be amazing!

ADVICE FOR BIRTH PARTNERS

The person giving birth is the most important person in the room.

During labour, they are often unable to communicate what they want and need.

This will be a time when you almost need to develop psychic skills in order to read what they are thinking or what they need. You are the messenger; you need to fight their corner, and make sure they've got what they need. Make sure that the music they want is on, that the lights are just so, that they have water/ice chips or a cold towel to wipe their forehead if they need it.

Don't keep asking them what they need; wait for them to ask you or just bring them something.

Asking somebody in labour lots of questions is just very overwhelming. It may be that what they normally find really comforting and enjoyable is not what they want in labour. Maybe they love a foot rub or a back rub or cuddles – but they might not want that in labour.

And above all, don't take anything personally.

This is an incredibly intense experience, so if they snap at you, or ignore you, just know that it's nothing to do with you; they're trying to get through this as best they can.

This will be a moment that neither of you will ever forget. You will talk about it for the rest of your lives.

SKIN-TO-SKIN – THE GOLDEN HOUR

If everything is fine with you and the baby, one of the first things that will happen after you give birth is that the midwife will put your baby onto your chest and suggest some skin-to-skin time to help you and your baby bond – ideally for around an hour at least, which is why it's referred to as 'the golden hour'. It's an important thing for the baby to feel safe and connected to you, and it's very important for you as a mother to feel connected to your baby.

Skin-to-skin contact means holding your newborn baby – naked or wearing only its nappy – against your bare chest, usually under a blanket so that you're both warm. Not only does it feel really lovely to hold your newborn directly against your skin, there is also mounting evidence to show that skin-to-skin contact has lots of other benefits. When your baby is on your chest and can hear the sound of your heartbeat and your voice, which is what it has heard for the last nine months, it feels reassured and safe. Skin-to-skin contact also helps:

— regulate your baby's temperature, breathing and heart rate

— prompt the release of oxytocin and other hormones to stimulate breastfeeding

— boost your milk supply if you're planning to breastfeed

— reduce your baby's stress levels

As I read more about the research behind skin to skin, I came across some fascinating information on the UNICEF UK website saying that skin-to-skin contact after birth initiates strong instinctive behaviours in both mum and baby. The mother will experience a surge of maternal hormones, while the baby's instincts will drive them to follow a unique process, which, if left uninterrupted, will cause them to have their first breastfeed. In other words, 'If they are enabled to familiarise themselves with their mother's breast and achieve self-attachment, it is very likely that they will recall this at subsequent feeds, resulting in fewer breastfeeding problems.'[45]

After birth, babies who are placed skin-to-skin on their mother's chest will:

— enter a stage of relaxation where they show very little movement as they recover from the birth

— start to wake up, opening their eyes and showing some response to mum's voice

— begin to make small movements of the arms, shoulders and head; as these movements increase, the baby will draw up their knees and appear to move or crawl towards the breast

— often rest once they have found the breast (this can often be mistaken for the baby not being hungry or not wanting to feed)

— begin to familiarise themselves with the breast after a period of rest, perhaps by nuzzling, smelling and licking around the area (this familiarisation period can last for some time and is important, so should not be rushed)

— self-attach and begin to feed (it may be that mum and baby need a little help with positioning at this stage)

— come off the breast once they have had a chance to suckle for a period of time. Following this, often both mother and baby will fall asleep[46]

What I found most fascinating about this was the point that babies often rest once they have found a breast, which can be mistaken for them not being hungry or not wanting to feed when that's not the case. Imagine: they've had to come out through a tiny birth canal and a vagina – they're exhausted, so of course they want to rest or just familiarise themselves with your breasts. Try to be patient and just allow the baby to work out how best to attach themselves. And then they'll come off the breast once they've had a chance to suckle for a bit.

I can relate to this strongly because with Holly, I was so nervous about her not latching on that I tried to stuff my nipple into her mouth the minute she came out. But she was so tired. She had been trying to be born for 36 hours and she was exhausted; she just needed to sleep for a little bit and then she would have found the boob when she was ready.

What I should have done was just keep her skin-to-skin and watch for when she was trying to nuzzle or find a nipple. What I ended up trying to do was forcing her to feed, and it made her a bit of a funny feeder for the first two weeks. With my next two, I was a bit more relaxed about trying to get them to breastfeed and just let them find my boob when they were ready. So, rather than doing what I did with Holly, let your baby root out your breast themselves.

Skin-to-skin contact after birth initiates strong instinctive behaviours in both mum and baby.

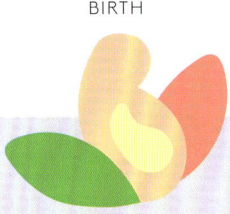

THE TESTS ONCE BABY IS BORN

Midwife Marley

One of the first things a midwife will do after the birth is ensure that both you and the baby are stable. Ideally, you should be able to experience some skin-to-skin time with your baby before they are examined and weighed – this promotes bonding and helps regulate the baby's temperature and heart rate. Immediately after birth, the first assessment of the baby is called the Apgar score. The Apgar score is used to assess the wellbeing of a baby at one minute, five minutes and, if necessary, ten minutes. The Apgar score looks at the following:

— **Appearance:** Is the baby pale and blue, or does the skin look normal and well perfused?

— **Pulse:** The baby's heart rate.

— **Grimace response:** Is the baby crying or making facial expressions? Are they responding to stimulation (reflexes)?

— **Activity (muscle tone):** Are they limp or are they moving their arms and legs?

— **Respiration:** Are they breathing at a normal rate?

The Apgar score is usually assessed while the baby is in the mother's arms. If the Apgar score is low (lower than seven), the baby may need to be taken across the room to a heated cot so that the midwife can help them a little. Most babies are born with very pale hands and feet. They may stay like this for a few days before changing to their normal colour.

The midwife will weigh the baby and check them over externally to make sure there are no obvious physical issues. The baby's temperature will be recorded, along with any birthmarks that have been observed.

If you have consented to your baby having vitamin K – an injection or oral solution to prevent vitamin K deficiency bleeding (VKDB) – this is given shortly after birth.

RECOVERY:
THE FIRST FEW HOURS

Everybody will feel a little bit different after they've given birth, depending on the kind of birth they've had. If you're feeling good and everything is fine, then the midwife will suggest skin-to-skin time to help you and the baby bond – I've gone into the benefits of this on page 217. I cannot stress enough what an amazing moment it is as you start to smell and nuzzle your baby and get to know each other. This is also a nice time for a partner to spend a bit of time skin-to-skin with the baby, too. But there are lots of other things that happen to your body after birth that you need to be aware of.

When I became a mother for the first time, nobody really spelled out to me what happens in the 24 hours after you've had a baby, or told me what was going to happen to my vagina. And, of course, it makes sense that if you have birthed a child, your vagina is going to need a little bit of TLC. When I say a little bit of TLC, actually there are quite a few things you can do to really help yourself. And you can start doing them almost immediately.

First off, you feel vulnerable down there. You feel swollen, you feel prolapsed – so, one of the things you want is compression, to make you feel held in. A great way of doing that is getting a snug pair of large underwear or compression pants, and you probably want three to four maternity pads in there. You may still be bleeding for about 24 hours after you've had a baby, and might even continue to bleed for about four or five weeks. When this happened to me, I kept thinking there was something wrong with me and didn't realise that it was actually quite normal. I did wear some quite snug compression pants, and that just helped make me feel safe.

You may also be experiencing pain as your uterus shrinks back down, which is referred to as afterpains. This starts happening naturally and, in fact, breastfeeding generally triggers it because the oxytocin it releases encourages the process – but it does mean you will experience discomfort. The pain is quite like period cramps, so a bit of warmth on your tummy, maybe from a hot-water bottle, can help soothe the area. I didn't find the pain too difficult to cope with, but if it's quite intense then do ask your midwife or a nurse for some pain relief.

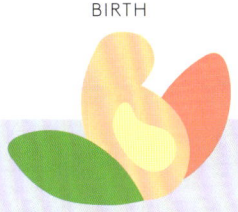

THE DIFFERENT TYPES OF RECOVERY

Midwife Marley

Your postnatal recovery journey begins as soon as you have given birth. The midwife will check that all your vital signs are okay, ensure you are not bleeding heavily and that the perineum has been sutured if necessary. If you have given birth in a hospital, a light meal/snack will be offered, and you will be able to shower, providing you haven't had an epidural and have full use of your legs. If you've had an epidural, the midwife will help to get you into clean clothes, and you'll be able to shower a bit later. Once you are stable and a bed is available, you'll be transferred to a postnatal ward. This could be anywhere from two to six hours after birth.

After a vaginal birth, your stay in hospital can last anywhere from six hours (if you've requested a quick discharge) to several days. It all depends on how you are healing after birth, and how the baby is doing. Most people who have had a caesarean will stay in hospital for at least one night. Before you are discharged home, a midwife will ensure you have all the essential information about birth registration, contact numbers for the hospital, the date of your first postnatal visit with the midwife, and information about contact with the health visitor and GP. If you have been prescribed any medication to take home, the midwife will go through all of this with you. They will want to make sure you are passing urine normally before discharging you, and that all your vital signs are normal. Before the baby is discharged, they will want to make sure they have passed urine and passed meconium (the baby's first poo), and that they are feeding well. When it's time to go home, somebody should be there to collect you, whether it's your birth partner, a family member, a friend or a taxi. Your baby should also have a car seat to be legal and safe to travel in a car.

If you have a home birth, the midwife will stay for some time after the birth and will only leave when they are happy that you and the baby are well. They will usually return the following day to check in on you.

Regardless of how and where you give birth, you should have an out-of-hours contact number in case any issues arise during the night when you are at home with your baby.

If you have had a caesarean, your postnatal journey will be different. Caesareans are major abdominal surgery, so the body needs time to fully recover. You'll spend time in recovery before being transferred to the postnatal ward. For many women, standing up after a caesarean doesn't happen for many hours, even until the next day if you give birth late in the afternoon or early evening. You'll need support from the maternity team and your birth partner to feed and care for your baby during your time in hospital after a caesarean.

It's not advised to lift anything heavier than your baby for a few weeks, and not to drive for six weeks. You will also need to check this with your insurance company. You may find that you have a lot of swelling in your hands and feet, and constipation post-birth is another common complaint. Drinking plenty of water may help with both of these. You may be prescribed compression socks to wear at home and blood-thinning injections to prevent blood clots. There is a risk of the wound becoming infected, so it is covered with a dressing for a few days until the midwife advises it be removed. Most

women will have sutures that are either dissolvable or will need removing in a few days. Occasionally staples are used to hold the wound together. Your midwife will advise you what type of wound closure has been used.

During those first hours after birth, you are likely to feel tired, sore and hungry! Don't hesitate to use the call buzzer on the ward if you need assistance.

'I ended up in hospital for five days [after birth] because I lost all sensation in my bladder.' — Sarah

I didn't know when I was weeing, and I needed to get that sorted. My baby needed me 24/7 while I was in the hospital, or so I thought. He wouldn't take a dummy; he would only take my little finger to suck on. I was struggling with breastfeeding; I was totally exhausted and not getting much sleep. I started to feel like I would not be able to look after my beautiful baby boy and really thought I would have to give him up. Luckily, one of the midwives saw the signs [of depression] and had a talk to me.

She simply said, 'You are not Super-mum. Your baby is demanding but let us help.' That night they took him to give me a rest and rest is what I did. I slept for the first time that night knowing my baby was in safe hands. Looking back, if I had left hospital within a day or so I would have undoubtedly ended up with postnatal depression. Instead, I listened to [the midwife's] advice, which helped me reset myself mentally, and when I left for home two days before Christmas, I let anyone who wanted to help, help.

Davina: Sarah, I am also one of those people that finds it incredibly hard to ask for help, but this is a fantastic example of why, when you have a baby, you absolutely need to take all the help you can get.

It is so important that as a new mum, you listen to your body and actively seek support because you're right: otherwise you might end up in a dark place and that's something we all want to try and avoid as much as we can.

WHAT IF THINGS DIDN'T GO ACCORDING TO YOUR BIRTH PLAN?

However much we prepare and plan for every eventuality, things won't always work out how we expected or wanted them to, and it can be very difficult to come to terms with this. Of course, there are different levels of disruption – you might have had to change your birth plan; you might have ended up in hospital when you'd planned to have a home birth; you might have had to have a C-section or there may have been unforeseen complications.

Whatever has happened to you, you may need support to move on and accept what's happened, or to prevent yourself becoming anxious or mentally stuck. If you have a partner, this is where they can step in; you will need to talk things through and support each other. If you don't have a partner, you will need to find somebody else to talk to. You will need to debrief. You might need to cry. You might need time to process what's happened. And please don't worry if you don't instantly feel the greatest love on earth for your baby – this could be because you have experienced birth trauma.

We've asked the brilliant Emma Mills, who is a specialist birth-trauma midwife, to talk about what this is, how you might be feeling, how to spot signs of trauma and where to go for help.

However much we prepare and plan for every eventuality, things won't always work out how we expected or wanted them to, and it can be very difficult to come to terms with this.

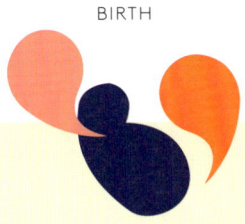

WHAT IS BIRTH TRAUMA?

Emma Mills, Midwife

The birth of your baby should be one of the most joyful days of your life, but it can be difficult to process these emotions when this is not your experience. One in four women in the UK find some part of the birth process traumatic, so it is essential to understand the feelings that arise as a result of experiencing trauma, the symptoms and how to access support.

Birth trauma relates not just to the physical, but also emotional experience of a distressing event that has occurred before, during or after childbirth. Many factors can increase the risk of birth trauma: an emergency during birth, excessive blood loss post-birth, medical intervention for you or your baby, your baby being taken away for a period of time or having a difficult feeding journey. Trauma can also be rooted in a lack of care you experienced, leaving you feeling helpless, unseen or unsafe. Any one of these factors can trigger the brain's survival mode, the 'fight/flight/freeze response', which your body activates when you perceive danger. This initiates a stress response in your body, and so you may feel very anxious,

uneasy, fearful or so overwhelmed you shut down, not remembering events that happened during your birth. This response can lead you to experiencing your birth as traumatic. Birth trauma is not only what happened; it is how you were left feeling.

You may not even recognise the trauma of your birth and are left struggling to enjoy your new family life and/or your next pregnancy without understanding why. You may feel trapped in negative thoughts, going over the birth in your mind, or feel unsafe. Ask yourself, do you:

— feel jumpy and startle easily?

— avoid talking about the birth to others?

— struggle to go to/stay asleep?

— avoid people you are close to?

— feel short-tempered or a sense of guilt?

— experience intrusive thoughts, nightmares or flashbacks?

If so, you may be experiencing symptoms of birth trauma. If you experience all of these symptoms for longer than a month, you may be diagnosed as suffering with post-traumatic stress disorder (PTSD). PTSD occurs when your brain is unable to deactivate your response to trauma and you are left in a constant state of hyperarousal, often experiencing the world around you as being very unsafe.

It can be hard to be honest about your feelings when there is a societal assumption that having a new baby is one of the most joyful times of your life. Acknowledging that you are struggling may be difficult, so you find it easier to say nothing. You may not even be aware that you are suffering from birth trauma for months, years or even until a next pregnancy.

It is not uncommon for birth trauma to also affect partners who have witnessed a traumatic birth, feared for the life of their partner and baby, felt unable to help their loved one or witnessed a lack of compassion or dignity in care.

If either you or your partner is struggling with the negative thoughts outlined above, please know that you are not alone. Recognising the symptoms and getting the right help is key. Having your questions answered, talking to your loved ones and being open about how you are feeling can help to process and manage your traumatic experience. Talk to your midwife, health visitor or GP, who may decide you would benefit from more support. They can refer you for talking therapies through the NHS, or more specialist services if they feel you may be experiencing PTSD. Alternatively, you can access a private birth-trauma therapist directly.

Birth trauma is an anxiety condition and is often confused with postnatal depression, which is a depressive condition. Unfortunately, women can be misdiagnosed with postnatal depression rather than birth trauma, and this can lead to incorrect treatment and a delay in recovery, impacting family life and relationships. Birth trauma can be treated, and you can heal from it. With the right help, you should be able to look back at the birth of your child without feeling a deep sense of fear, panic or guilt, allowing you and your partner to move forward and enjoy your family.

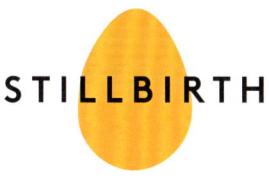

STILLBIRTH

Losing a baby, whether though miscarriage, stillbirth or following its birth, is unimaginable and I cannot begin to know the right words to comfort those of you who have had to go through such a devastating experience.

Marley is going to explain below what happens when a baby is stillborn, and then the amazing Heather has so bravely shared her experience of baby loss, which we hope will help anyone else who has to navigate the same grief and heartache.

WHAT HAPPENS WHEN A BABY IS STILLBORN?

Marley: A stillbirth occurs when a baby sadly dies after 24 weeks of pregnancy before they are born. It is a devastating event that happens in around 1 in 250 pregnancies in the UK. Some are linked to problems with the placenta, or anomalies within the baby or the mother's health. Quite often, the cause is simply unknown.

Many stillbirths are detected when cessation of foetal movements have been reported in pregnancy, and an ultrasound scan confirms no heartbeat. It is not common for a baby to pass away during labour.

When it has been confirmed that a baby has died, the mother may be able to wait for labour to occur, or she may prefer to be induced. Stillborn babies are rarely born by caesarean.

After the birth of the baby, the parents can spend time with and hold the baby if they wish. The midwife may arrange for hand-/footprints, and you will be able to take photographs. Women who experience a stillbirth are not placed on a postnatal ward with other mums and babies; they will be able to spend time with their baby in a private room before being discharged home when they are stable enough. Further tests may be carried out to identify the cause of death, but this will be discussed with the parents beforehand. Before leaving the hospital, the parents will be given information about birth and death registration, postnatal visits and support services. Once the death has been registered, the parents are then able to think about burial or cremation. The hospital is usually able to organise this with the parents, but some parents prefer to organise it themselves.

A stillborn baby may invoke feelings of grief, confusion, guilt and anger – all are completely normal. The chance of postnatal depression is also increased in those who have experienced a stillbirth, as the body will go through all the changes that would occur with a live baby. Experiencing these things without a baby can make it more difficult to cope with.

Many hospitals will have a bereavement specialist midwife, and there are other independent services that can offer support, such as Sands (Stillbirth and Neonatal Death Society), and Tommy's charity.

There is no right or wrong way to navigate loss. Some parents will want to talk about it and others won't. Some parents will find the initial grieving period very difficult and lengthy, and others won't. The period of grief after losing a baby has no time limit.

YOUR STORIES

'I found the first few months of pregnancy quite straightforward until one morning I had a midwife appointment and everything changed.' — Heather

I remember I was tired after working, so when my midwife calmly said she had to make a phone call to the hospital to

check something, I didn't think anything of it. Before I knew it, I was heading to hospital with an overnight bag just in case. I was admitted and had a number of tests, then was told I needed to stay in overnight for monitoring.

When my husband arrived in the morning we saw the consultant. He informed us that I had pre-eclampsia [see page 144] and HELLP syndrome [see page 145] and I was extremely poorly. This was a massive shock as I felt fine. Over the next few hours we had numerous conversations with the consultant, which ended in him informing us that if we didn't deliver our baby, my husband could lose both of us. I was only 24 weeks and 5 days, so the risk of our baby dying was high. I still couldn't believe what I was hearing as I didn't feel that unwell. They were becoming more and more concerned by my condition so we had to make the difficult decision for them to induce labour, knowing there was a high possibility that our little girl would be stillborn.

At 6.30 p.m. I gave birth to a beautifully formed tiny little girl and our nightmare came true. She was born sleeping. After labour, my condition instantly improved, and although we were devastated, I could see the relief on my husband's face that I was out of danger.

The days and nights that followed are still a blur. The thing I can remember was how amazing the hospital staff were, giving us time to spend with our beautiful girl and say goodbye to her. Despite having to go through labour and holding our tiny baby in our arms, we weren't officially allowed to register her. We were blessed to be able to have a funeral and say a proper goodbye, which was a little unusual as I wasn't quite 25 weeks and at that time officially her

birth couldn't be registered as a stillbirth. Telling people was hard, and seeing how they struggled to respond was harder.

Thankfully we have been since blessed with two beautiful healthy children, who are now adults, but for years I found it hard to deal with people's response [to our loss] so would say I had two children, breaking my heart every time and wanting to shout, 'Actually, I have three children.' Twenty-six years have passed and now, if people ask me, I don't care how they respond: I have three children but unfortunately our first little girl was stillborn. I am mum to three children and that will never change. Writing this down after all this time feels amazing, and if our story helps just one parent come to terms with their loss and feel able to talk about their baby, then we are glad we shared our story.

Davina: Heather, I am so grateful to you for having the courage and the generosity to tell us your story. I know that your account of your experience will help other women going through something similar and navigate what must be the toughest of times. Thank you so very much.

'The pregnancy progressed in exactly the same way as my first one did – all-day sickness from hell but always with an overwhelming feeling of excitement.' — Cathy

The 20-week scan was booked for a Friday morning. We took our 5-year-old daughter to the scan, planning to drop her at school afterwards.

When a sonographer goes quiet and says 'there's a problem', gets up to leave the room and comes back with someone to give a second opinion – instinct tells you it's not good!

Mark took our daughter outside and I waited alone and after whispered conversations heard the news that our baby had a hole in its heart.

The scan was on a Friday morning and we were told no more investigations could be done until the Monday and we were sent home. The next few weeks were full of referrals, appointments, scans, blood tests and amniocentesis (to check for Down's syndrome which was the most likely cause for heart babies). The amniocentesis wasn't an easy decision – we were warned it came with a risk of miscarriage but were advised it was the right thing to do so we went ahead. We are also advised on many occasions that a termination was an option – for me it never was but it did prompt uncomfortable conversations between us both.

We were referred to St George's for scans and monitoring and eventually had our appointment with a leading heart specialist and someone who I will never forget for his kindness and going above and beyond when everyone was ready to give up. The scans turned out to be spot on – our baby had four major heart abnormalities. They had seen all four before but never in the same baby; the odds of having all these issues together were the same chances as winning the lottery!

The plan was surgery on her first day in the world to buy some time and then a heart transplant if we were lucky enough to get one (a transplant was bittersweet because for us to save our baby, we knew someone else would need to lose theirs, so we needed to navigate those emotions on top of everything else).

We were warned that if we did get as far as 39/40 weeks and managed to give birth, she would be born blue and would need intervention immediately and only at that point would they know if her *lungs had developed enough to take her own first breath.*

I went through the pregnancy with positivity, not allowing myself to focus on the worst-case scenario or the detail, drawing on all the letters of love we received. She did survive to term and at 38 weeks I went into labour at our local hospital in south London. Royal Brompton were alerted that a bed would be needed later that night for the transfer.

On 17 February Macey was born and let out the biggest cry. She didn't need any interactions – her lungs had developed, the relief was palpable. The tears flowed and she was handed to me for a cuddle. I felt nervous to hold her for too long and just wanted them to get her into the incubator and down to the paediatric intensive care unit (PICU) to see how she was.

Once ready, Mark and I sat looking at her in the incubator with wires all over her body and splints wrapped in bandages on her hands to stop her pulling any wires off while she was checked over and a plan made for her transfer. The consultant was amazed at how well she looked.

Macey was blue lighted to Great Ormond Street as no beds were available at the Royal Brompton. A midwife left me in my hospital room at midnight; it was one of the loneliest nights of my life. The following morning I discharged myself. My dad came up to collect me with my daughter and we made the uncomfortable journey up to Great Ormond Street.

On 1 March we had to make the agonising decision to turn off Macey's

life support machine (no transplant heart had been found and her health had deteriorated so much it meant she wouldn't have survived the operation). I could not bring myself to say 'goodbye' but did kiss her forehead and hold her hand. I didn't want her to think I'd given in and accepted her death and somehow saying goodbye felt too final.

My plan has always been to try and write a book of hope and positivity to keep Macey's memory alive and for her to be spoken about in the present tense – to show others that life does carry on and resume some normality even for those of us that don't get the outcomes we deserve.

Davina: Cathy, thank you for telling me about Macey. She sounds absolutely amazing, and I love the idea of a book.

In the meantime, I know that the fact that you and Mark are able to share Macey's story will really make a difference to others. We are so grateful to you both.

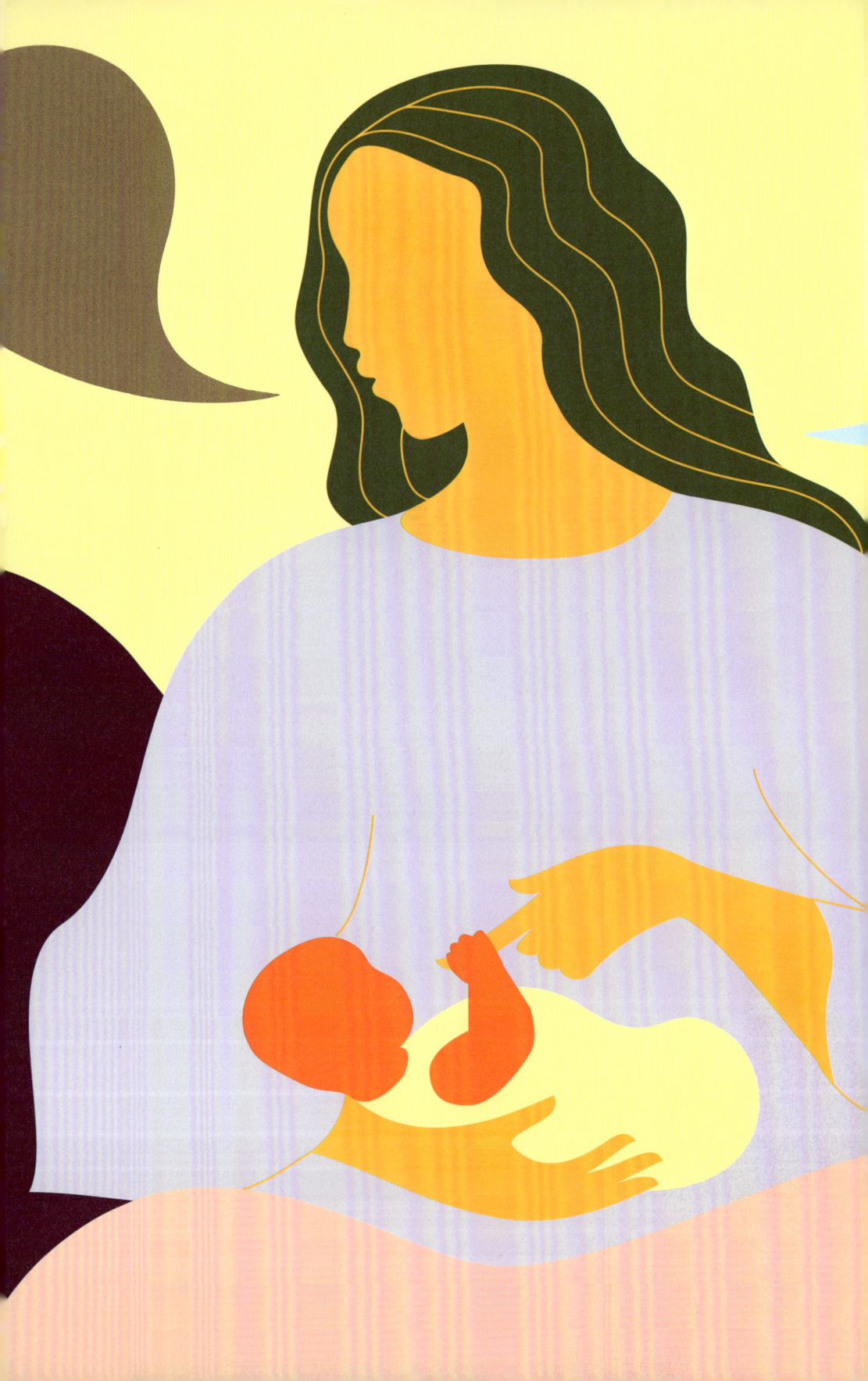

CHAPTER 6

FOURTH TRIMESTER/ POSTPARTUM

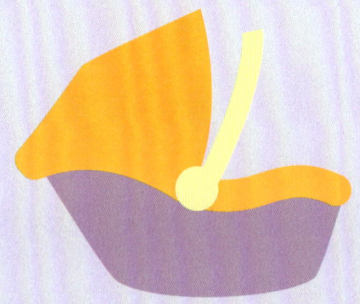

Trust your instincts...

LIFE WITH A NEWBORN

Those first few hours, days and weeks after you give birth are such a jumble of emotions: excitement, exhaustion, trepidation, unbridled joy, and disbelief that you carried the tiny person in front of you for nine months and now they're here.

My midwife stayed the night with me after my first birth, and when she did leave the next day, I remember wanting to cling on to her for dear life and beg her to stay. But she told me I was going to be fine and that I knew what I was doing. 'Listen to yourself. And trust your instincts,' she said. Looking back now, I think that was a good reminder that in modern society we don't often do that. We're constantly bombarded with information and often conflicting advice, which means that we've lost confidence in our ability to trust ourselves and follow our gut. And I am grateful to Pam for saying it to me because it stuck with me, and she was right – a mother's instinct is usually correct; you just KNOW when something's off. I could always tell when any of my children weren't quite right. But her leaving me and walking out the door, and it just being us left at home, was at once such a strange and overwhelming feeling, and yet somehow the most natural thing in the world. I changed in that moment because I was holding this little person whose life I would now forever put before my own.

I love the old adage, 'It takes a village to raise a child.' In this day and age, we can all be so far away from each other, which means it can be difficult for new parents to get the family support that was once taken for granted. There used to be an understanding that we would all learn to parent from our own parents and grandparents, and that they would be there to support us on our parenting journey. But these days that just isn't always physically – or emotionally – feasible. When I gave birth, my mum and I were on shaky ground and my dad and stepmum were living in Portsmouth and I was living in Surrey, which is quite a trek. But I was extremely lucky to have some amazing next-door neighbours called Mandy and Greg, who lived a five-minute walk away. They literally became my lifeline. Holly went through a stage of waking up at 5 a.m. every morning and I would start to count the minutes until 7 a.m. when I could walk down to Mandy's with her and have breakfast or a cup of tea.

Postpartum – or the fourth trimester, as it's also known – describes the first three to six months after a baby is born. Your baby is learning to adjust to its new world, and you are navigating a maelstrom of physical and mental changes as your body recovers from everything it was put through during pregnancy and birth. Your hormones are going crazy, you're suddenly having to adjust to life with a lot less sleep and you're confronting a lot of emotions. In this chapter, we've tried to cover what to expect and how you can thrive during this time, or where you can turn for the support and guidance we all need as we navigate the shift into motherhood.

235

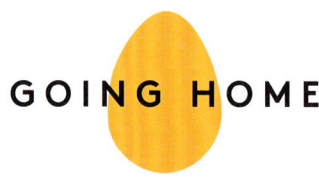

GOING HOME

Leaving the hospital will throw up such a mixture of emotions. You might be an excited new mum doing this incredible thing on your own, or if you're becoming a parent with a partner, you may both be feeling so happy and proud because you went into that hospital as two, and you've come out as three, four or, in a friend of mine's case, five. But this moment may also not be what you'd planned at all – you might be feeling anxious, depressed or frightened; you may be having to leave your baby in the hospital's care, or you might have suffered the trauma of another complication. If that is the case, then please, please reach out for help using the resources we've provided (see page 308). And, of course, even if everything has gone to plan, it's also an incredibly nerve-racking time, and I want to remind you that that's normal and okay. You're on your own with this little newborn – you're responsible for it and that can feel daunting. You are also going to be very tired. If you've asked for a quick discharge, it will only be six hours since you gave birth, and so you want to take it very easy.

If you're going home by car, one of the first practical steps is to get your baby into its car seat. I cannot stress enough how helpful it is to have practised this ad infinitum in the weeks running up to the birth. You want to learn how the seat clips into the car because sometimes it's difficult, and if you have a partner, make sure they've practised it, too. You should also make sure you've brought the car seat into the hospital in plenty of time and that you settle the baby into it in the warmth indoors, because if it's winter and you've just brought the seat inside from a cold car, you'll be putting the baby into a freezing car seat and that will make them cry, which will make you very upset and stressed.

The great thing about nesting (see page 136) is that, hopefully, you already have everything you and your baby need for the next few days and weeks, so when you get home, once your partner or somebody else has helped you get the car seat indoors, the only thing you need to do is get into a pair of comfy PJs and settle into bed or a comfy spot on the sofa to rest. You want to make sure you've got everything close to you so that you don't have to get up and move around. Have water, snacks, nappies, muslins, any medication you're taking and your phone charger close by – preferably in a box right next to you.

It can be quite a good idea to bring a mini-kettle nearer to you if you're staying in your bedroom, so that you don't have to go downstairs or walk too far to have a cup of tea or coffee.

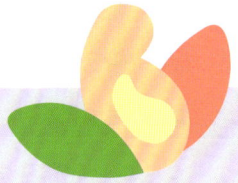

FIRST MEDICAL VISITS

Midwife Marley

A midwife will routinely be in contact the day after you leave the hospital/birth centre, or the day after a home birth. They will also see you on around days five and ten after the birth, often in a community setting like a GP surgery. Additional contact may be necessary from the midwife or infant-feeding specialist if there are any issues that arise postnatally or if feeding support is required. Around day ten, all being well, your care is transferred over to the local health visitors, who will be attached to you and your family until your baby is five years old. They will be the ones to contact with queries about immunisations and child development.

During postnatal visits, the midwife will ask you questions about your recovery – whether you're eating and drinking okay, and what your blood loss is like. They may ask to check stitches if you have had any perineal tears, or your caesarean wound if you've had one. Postnatal visits are a good time to talk about how you're feeling. The first few days can be a bit of a rollercoaster, with feelings ranging from elation, to tiredness and feeling weepy. Your

midwife will want to support you both mentally and physically during this time.

Your baby will be weighed around day five, and most babies will have lost a bit of weight, more so if they are breastfed. This is normal and is impacted by things like fluids given during labour, and the fact that colostrum takes a few days to change into full milk that increases in volume. A loss of up to 10 per cent of birth weight can be considered normal.

A test called newborn blood spot screening (NBSS) is offered around day five to all babies in the UK by pricking the baby's heel and taking several spots of blood onto a special paper. It screens for a variety of metabolic, endocrine and blood disorders, along with cystic fibrosis. The test is then sent off to a national screening lab to be checked.

There can be a lot to take in during the first few days, so, where possible, have someone with you for support. You may want to mark important things like appointments in your diary. The postnatal period can make you forgetful, particularly if you are exhausted.

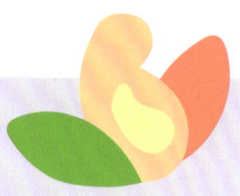

YOUR BODY
AND ITS RECOVERY

Midwife Marley

The body goes through a number of changes that can be quite surprising but are totally normal as you recover from pregnancy and birth.

The uterus spends a couple of weeks contracting down to pre-pregnancy size. During this time, there will be some blood loss from the vagina. Bleeding may be heavy at first and then settle, only to appear heavier again from time to time, particularly on exertion. This is why listening to your body and resting when you can is so important. If bleeding becomes very heavy all of a sudden and you are completely soaking through pads in less than an hour, contact your maternity unit for advice. Small blood clots are normal, but any that are larger than a satsuma, or that are accompanied by excessive bleeding, should be reported to the midwife.

If you feel afterpains and cramps in your uterus, applying pressure with a warm flannel or towel could be beneficial. You might find that other parts of your body, like the thighs, will ache a little, too. After some rest, bodily aches do go away.

Perineal discomfort is common, particularly if you have had stitches. These will heal over the coming weeks but keeping the area clean and dry in the meantime is essential. Avoid using perfumed soaps when bathing or showering. It may be sore when passing urine, which can be alleviated by pouring a bottle of warm water onto the area while you're on the toilet. To offer even more comfort, you might wish to try a postpartum relief spray. After a week or so, if you had stitches, you might notice that the sutures are coming out. This indicates that the injury is beginning to mend. Do let your healthcare practitioner know if your pain seems to be getting worse every day.

You can have sensitive, swollen breasts a few days after birth due to the change and increase of milk volume. We will talk more about breastfeeding further in the book, but it's good to know that this swelling, called engorgement, is only temporary. A good-fitting bra, regular feeding and a cold compress may help alleviate discomfort. It's common to go up a cup size or two during pregnancy, so make sure your bra isn't digging in, but that your breasts are feeling well supported. Many stores will have a bra-fitting service that you can utilise if you are unsure of your size. Non-underwired bras are more comfortable postnatally but there are many options for nursing/maternity bras, which allow for easy access to the breasts when you are feeding your baby.

Other, less spoken-about postnatal symptoms include night sweats and headaches. Night sweats are temporary while the hormones try to regulate themselves. Any headaches experienced are usually mild, temporary and alleviated with plenty of hydration and paracetamol. Persistent headaches should be reported to your maternity unit.

If you are experiencing difficult feelings or if you think your partner is a bit detached, please let the midwife know.

Sometimes, if a new mother is having ongoing physical or psychological issues, it really is down to a partner or loved one to notice this.

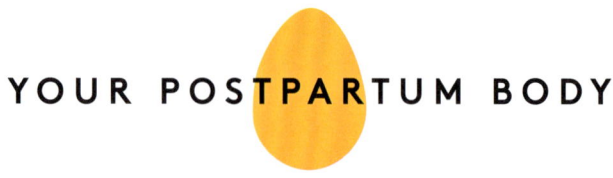

YOUR POSTPARTUM BODY

Jenny Gillespie, a specialist pelvic health physiotherapist, has outlined below some of the details of the recovery process your body will be going through, depending on what kind of birth you had. She will also cover when and how to start pelvic-floor exercises, which is something you want to start thinking about fairly early on. I cannot stress enough how important Jenny's advice is! I remember I used to pee like a racehorse before I had babies. After I had babies, that really changed. And the pelvic-floor exercises are vital. If, later in life, you would like to have better control of your pelvic floor and not be somebody who has to cross their legs immediately if somebody tells a really funny joke, then starting your exercises early on is a really, really good idea.

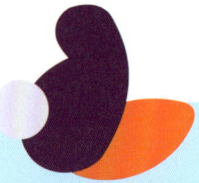

EARLY POSTPARTUM RECOVERY

Jenny Gillespie, Specialist Pelvic Health Physiotherapist

Your baby has arrived! There is a lot to take in and everything may feel a bit overwhelming. It is important to give yourself time and permission to heal. There is so much pressure on mums to get back to 'normal' and do everything as soon as possible. Your body has been amazing, growing and birthing a baby, but it has also undergone some changes that need time and care to heal. Everyone's attention will naturally be focused on the new arrival, but it is essential that you and your needs are prioritised, too. Please do not expect to

be completely back to normal –
physically or emotionally – by the time
you have your postnatal GP check-up
at six weeks (you may be, but don't
worry if you're not).

VAGINAL DELIVERY

If you have delivered your baby vaginally,
your perineum and vagina will have
stretched to allow the baby to be born.
These can take some time to return to
normal and the area may feel sore and
swollen for the first couple of weeks.

You may have been given an episiotomy,
or the perineum may have torn during
delivery. These tears are graded
according to which parts of the
perineum are involved (see page 195).
There can also be damage to the
pelvic-floor muscles, which can lead
to issues like incontinence, pain
and prolapse.[47]

All perineal injuries can be sore as
they heal. Look after them by washing
with clear water only and drying fully,
changing pads regularly, sitting on a
cushion, applying ice packs for pain
and swelling, and taking painkillers
if required.

Once the scar is fully healed it can help
to touch and gently massage the area.
Movement can improve blood flow to
the area and help form a soft, mobile
scar that is less restricted. Simple
exercises like pelvic tilts or cat stretch
can help with pain and moving the
scar tissue.

It is safe to start pelvic-floor exercises
as soon as you are comfortable. The
muscles may feel weak and you may
not feel much of a contraction initially,
especially if you have had a traumatic
delivery, but persevere and it
will improve.

If you feel a significant increase in pain
that doesn't settle within an hour of
doing any type of exercise, this may be
too much at this stage of your recovery
and you may need to progress more
slowly. This shouldn't be the case with
pelvic-floor exercises. If they do cause
you pain, please see your GP.

CAESAREAN SECTION

If you deliver by C-section, all of the
above advice applies. A caesarean
section is major abdominal surgery.
You may need to take a little more
time to rest and recover. Pelvic-floor
exercises are just as important
following a caesarean delivery, as
although it is not exposed to the
stretch and direct trauma of vaginal
birth, your pelvic floor has still had
to adapt to the postural and weight
changes that occur during pregnancy
and therefore needs rehabilitation.

EARLY SCAR MANAGEMENT

There is a lot that you can do in the early days to support effective healing and formation of a healthy C-section scar:

— Hydration and nutrition are important for good scar healing.

— Once the dressing is removed, wash only with clear water and pat dry with a clean towel.

— Allow time for the scar to 'breathe', leaving it uncovered for short periods.

— If any areas open up, if the scar becomes red, hot or swollen, or if there is any oozing, please see your GP.

— As soon as you feel able, it is beneficial to start to 'engage' with your scar. This can be difficult for some people, especially if there is trauma associated with their delivery. It is an important step to accepting your birth experience and starting your recovery. Take your time. It can initially be just looking at your scar using a mirror. Then progress to touching your tummy and the area around the scar, moving onto the scar itself. Engaging with your scar helps you re-establish a connection with your tummy that may have been lost after a traumatic delivery. It can help improve sensation by stimulating the nerve endings and be a good step towards starting scar massage.

Once the scar has fully healed and your stitches are removed or have dissolved, you can start scar massage. You should wait four to six weeks after your C-section, and it is best to have been checked by your GP, nurse or physiotherapist before starting to massage your scar. Scar massage can help the blood flow and sensation around the scar, improving the mobility of the scar and surrounding tissue, which can lead to a more comfortable scar that doesn't pull when you move.[48] Spend a couple of minutes on each step and build up at your own speed to complete all the steps.

Step 1: Get into a comfortable position where you can easily touch your scar. This is usually lying down with your head supported on a pillow.

Step 2: Start by gently touching your tummy and the area around the scar with a light, sweeping motion using the flat of your hand. Take your time. If this is all you are happy doing in the early days, you can progress to more specific massage over the scar when you are ready.

Step 3: When you are ready to move on, you can start touching above, below and directly on the scar with the tip of your finger. Note if any areas feel tender, tight, bumpy or numb. Keep the tip of your finger in contact with the skin and move the finger forwards, backwards and in small circles as you move along the length of the scar.

Step 4: Holding one end of the scar with one finger, slide the finger of the other hand a few centimetres along the scar. Move the first finger to meet the second, brace and slide again. Work left to right and back again along the scar.

Step 5: Brace the scar with one finger (of the same hand) either side of it. You can move the index finger of the other hand across the scar in a zigzag pattern or slide your finger up and down over the scar.

Step 6: Finally, you can try rolling your scar. Taking two fingers, try moving areas of your scar up towards your head and down towards your toes. Some areas of your scar may feel more restricted than others. You can also try with the fingers of one hand above and one hand below, bringing the two sides of the scar together and lifting slightly, working along the length of the scar.

If you would like to use an oil for your scar massage, it is best to choose one that specifies it is for scar massage. You can perform the techniques above without oil.

If your scar is raised or keloid (bumpy, thickened and raised scars), these need special attention. You can still massage above and below the scar and move and roll it, but direct pressure and friction over the scar should be light. The gold-standard treatment for raised and keloid scars is silicone. There are many different products on the market, including gels that you can massage into the skin, and silicone-infused stick-on strips that can be left in place for several hours. For the best results, you should choose a product with medical-grade silicone.

COMMON POSTNATAL PELVIC-FLOOR PROBLEMS (AND WHAT YOU CAN DO ABOUT THEM)

Incontinence

You may start to notice that some things do not feel quite the same as they did before pregnancy. How many times have you heard a mum say there's no way she could jump on a trampoline without wetting herself? Although it is very common, especially after having a baby, urinary incontinence is definitely NOT something you need to put up with! Leaking can either be due to stress incontinence, which is when you leak urine under pressure (coughing, sneezing, laughing, lifting or running), or urge incontinence, which is needing to wee suddenly, being unable to hold on or leaking just before getting to the loo.

Some women experience faecal incontinence – they leak from their bowel, which is particularly common if there was a third- or fourth-degree tear;[49] they may also have difficulty controlling wind.

Any type of incontinence is usually due to the pelvic-floor muscles not working at their best following pregnancy and birth. They can be weak, lack endurance (the ability to work well over a period of time), or they can actually be overactive and not fully relaxing. The latter is actually very common. If the muscles hold tension and don't relax, they can't work as well as if they contract from a relaxed position. They may also fatigue more quickly. It's important to understand how to activate your pelvic floor correctly.

Top tips if you are experiencing incontinence include the following:

— Stay hydrated but stick to clear water and herbal teas. Avoid anything that may irritate the bladder and make you want to wee more often. This could be caffeine, alcohol, diet fizzy drinks and fruit juices.

— Empty your bladder regularly (every three to four hours). Try not to go when you don't really need to or 'just in case'. This will help train the bladder to be able to hold a normal volume of urine.

— Take your time on the loo. You may need to rock forwards and backwards or change positions to make sure you have fully emptied your bladder.

— Avoid constipation. This can put the pelvic floor under a lot of strain. Stay hydrated and eat lots of fruit and vegetables. If you feel you need to strain, sit on the toilet with your feet up on a stool (so your knees are higher than your hips) and take some deep breaths to relax the pelvic floor. Try not to push or bear down. If this doesn't work, speak to your GP.

— Practise pelvic-floor exercises to improve the function of the muscles (see page 246).[50]

— Ask to be referred to a pelvic health physiotherapist for more help.

Pelvic organ prolapse (POP)

Another common symptom can be a feeling of heaviness or dragging in the pelvis or a sensation of bulging in the vagina. This may feel like a tampon that is not inserted correctly. Often this feeling happens during activities like walking, as you are starting to do a little bit more or when lifting. It can get worse towards the end of the day but feel better after rest or in the morning.

These symptoms can just be part of the normal healing process, particularly if there is swelling or trauma to the muscles, and they can improve within the first six weeks postpartum. It is possible, however, that they may be signs of a pelvic organ prolapse.

Your bladder, bowel and uterus are supported in the pelvis by the pelvic-floor muscles and a system of connective tissue. This system can be affected by postural and weight changes in pregnancy as well as stretch and trauma during delivery, resulting in either the bladder, bowel or uterus dropping down into the vagina. This can be made worse when the pressure in your abdomen and pelvis increases (intra-abdominal pressure) during activities like lifting, coughing and jumping. The best way to check if this is the case is to have a vaginal examination by a GP, gynaecologist or specialist physiotherapist.

The most common types of prolapse are:

— **Cystocele:** The bladder and front wall of the vagina descend.

— **Rectocele:** The rectum and back wall of the vagina descend.

— **Uterine:** The uterus descends.

Risk factors for prolapse include being overweight, chronic constipation, a traumatic vaginal delivery (especially with the use of forceps), a third- or fourth-degree tear, a family history of POP and hypermobility syndromes.

As well as the heaviness or bulging sensation, you may also have problems with incontinence or difficulty fully emptying your bladder or bowel. Some people experience discomfort or changes in sensation when having sex.

POP can seriously affect a new mother's mental health and body image, and can be very frightening. It is important to know that with the right help, symptoms can be managed well. Although it is difficult to say whether it will resolve completely, in the postnatal period recovery is ongoing and there are still lots of hormonal changes occurring. Time and the right management will often lead to an improvement in symptoms.

Below are some top tips for managing prolapse:

— Start your pelvic-floor exercises as soon as you are comfortable with movement (see page 290).[51]

— Lift objects correctly and manage your abdominal pressure. Breathe out and engage your core and pelvic-floor muscles as you lift.

— Avoid constipation (as explained above).

— Practise good bladder habits and hydration (as explained above).

— Build in sit-down rest periods as you increase your activity levels.

— Take care if using a baby sling. These can increase POP symptoms and should be used for short periods and ideally not when you are experiencing symptoms.

— See a pelvic health physiotherapist. They will be able to assess your prolapse and help you progress your pelvic-floor training and manage your symptoms. They may also talk to you about a pessary, which is a silicone device inserted into the vagina to support the walls and reduce your symptoms.

PELVIC-FLOOR EXERCISES – HOW DO YOU DO THEM?

If you went to a new gym class, it's likely that the instructor would teach you how to perform the exercises involved and check if your technique was correct. That's a bit trickier with the pelvic floor as it's not visible, so lots of people are not sure if they are doing the exercises correctly. Follow the steps below to guide you:

Step 1: Start off in a comfortable position: lying on your back or your side with a cushion under your knees is easiest to start with.

Step 2: Begin by taking a few slow breaths in and out, allowing the lower ribs to expand in all directions like a balloon inflating. Try to breathe in for a count of three and out for six. This will help you fully utilise your diaphragm (the breathing muscle), which in turn helps the pelvic floor to lift and lower. Try to visualise your pelvic-floor muscles releasing as you gently breathe in.

Step 3: When you are ready, you can start the pelvic-floor contractions. As you breathe out, think about tightening the muscles around your back passage (as if you were trying to stop wind escaping) and draw those muscles up inside you and forwards towards your belly button. Try to keep your bottom and hip muscles as relaxed as possible.

Step 4: Hold the contraction if you can for five to ten seconds and fully release. It's okay to have a rest in between contractions; you don't have to go on every breath.

Aim for three sets of ten repetitions daily, but you may have to build up to this in the early days.

Once you're comfortable with these exercises, you can try quicker contractions where you lift and then fully release. A good tool for tracking your pelvic-floor exercises is the Squeezy App (thesqueezyapp.com).

Once you have mastered these exercises lying down, it is really important to start practising them sitting, standing and eventually during activities like squatting and lifting. This is more challenging but also more functional. Few people leak lying down!

Don't feel embarrassed about asking for help with these symptoms. You can ask to be referred to a specialist pelvic health physiotherapist by your GP. You can also find a list of practitioners working near you by visiting: thepogp.co.uk.

Other postnatal conditions a physiotherapist can help with include:

— diastasis recti (separation of the abdominal muscles)

— painful sex

— lower back, hip or ongoing pelvic pain

— support with returning to exercise.

Your physiotherapist will ask questions about your pregnancy and birth, and any symptoms you may be experiencing. They will then undertake a thorough assessment of your posture and how you move. They will be able to check your abdominal muscles for a gap or diastasis and check how your abdominal and core muscles are recovering. If you have had a perineal tear or C-section, they will assess your scar and give you advice on caring for it. Finally, if you are happy to, they may perform an internal vaginal examination. This is to check for prolapse and to assess the function of the pelvic-floor muscles. It is quick and usually painless, and can be used to check that you know how to perform pelvic-floor exercises correctly.

Your physiotherapist can offer advice, education, exercises, scar therapy and other hands-on treatment to help you recover from your birth and address all of the issues discussed above. Don't put up with these uncomfortable, distressing symptoms. There is lots of support to regain your health and strength in your journey as a mum.

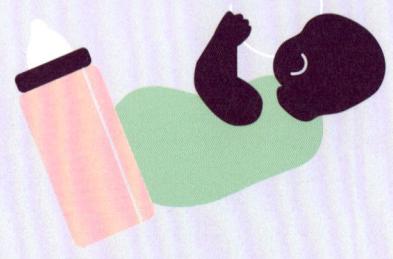

FEEDING

Midwife Marley

Infant feeding has become a hugely controversial topic, with thousands of people sharing their opinions and stories online. One thing we can mostly agree on is that the way in which you decide to feed your baby is a personal choice. The views of those around us can have an impact on decisions we make regarding feeding our babies. It can be difficult to block out the noise, so this section is designed to give you as much information as possible to help you understand infant feeding.

Babies need to have milk for at least the first year of life. Milk should be an exclusive part of their diet for the first six months, and comes in the form of either breastmilk or formula milk. The World Health Organization (WHO) recommends exclusive breastfeeding for the first six months, and continuing to breastfeed in combination with solid foods and water for two years and beyond if both mother and baby wish.

In the UK, approximately 68 per cent of people start breastfeeding, with only 48 per cent still doing so at the six-to-eight-week mark. There are lots of reasons for this, including lack of support, difficulties with feeding due to things like tongue tie, mums feeling like their baby isn't getting enough milk, pressure from family members who want to feed the baby, returning early to work and complications such as mastitis.

BREASTFEEDING

Breastfeeding is known to have several benefits for both mother and baby, including:

— Lower chance of the baby developing infections.

— Reduced incidence of diarrhoea and vomiting (gastroenteritis) in babies.

— Lower chance of SIDS (sudden infant death syndrome).

— Lower chance of the baby developing heart disease later in life.

— Lower chance of obesity, probably due to babies being better able to regulate their food intake from the breast, and improvement in their gut health.

— Lower chance of breast and ovarian cancer for mums.

— Lower chance of osteoporosis later in life for mums.

— Feeding from the breast saves time, the milk is the right temperature, and it's free.

Breastfeeding, although the biological norm, doesn't come easily or naturally to everyone. If you decide to breastfeed your baby, understanding the process and seeking help and support before you start will increase your chances of success. Before your baby arrives, it might be a good idea to attend a breastfeeding class, unless the topic is covered in any antenatal courses you may have enrolled with. Find out if there are any local breastfeeding support groups and the contact details for the hospital's infant-feeding team, in case you need them.

Understanding the physiology of breastmilk is crucial, as it's easy to assume you don't have enough milk in the early days before the colostrum (see page 151) changes into 'full milk'. After birth, it's ideal for the baby to feed within its first hour, and this first feed tends to be a lengthy one. The midwife will help you with this. After the first feed, the baby may sleep for a long time before wanting to feed again. Babies often only feed a handful of times in the first 24 hours as they recover from being born, but this usually changes after the first day. Over the coming days, it's normal for them to want to feed often, sometimes every two hours, sometimes flitting between one and three hours. Sometimes it feels as though they are constantly feeding to encourage the milk to 'come in' quicker. There is no set time between feeds, and midwives encourage something called 'responsive feeding'. When a baby shows signs they are hungry, offer the breast, even if it's only been a short time since the last feed. Signs that your baby might be hungry include sucking their fingers or fists, rooting with their mouths, wriggling and rapid eye movements. These usually occur before the baby starts to cry.

The amount of colostrum that the baby gets each feed is small, just a few millilitres at a time. It's unlikely you will see much of it, which can make some people feel anxious as to whether there is actually any there! The midwife will observe the baby to ensure they don't appear dehydrated, and wet/dirty nappies will also help to alleviate any concerns. As the milk changes and increases in volume around day five to six, the baby's poo increases and turns yellow, indicating that they are getting enough milk. When breastfeeding, you should be aiming to drink around 3 litres of water a day, and make sure you are eating adequately. If you've harvested colostrum during your pregnancy, this can be given to your baby at any point, as long as it hasn't been in the freezer past the recommended six months. It's beneficial at any time.

CHALLENGES WITH BREASTFEEDING

I always advise parents to have the contact details for breastfeeding support in case they face any difficulties. It's not uncommon for feeding to go well on the first day, and then for problems with latching on to arise once you get home. Engorged breasts are often the culprit, as a baby may find it difficult latching on to them, so hand-expressing a small amount of milk before attempting to latch baby on may be necessary. Breastfeeding in general shouldn't be painful. That said, if the baby isn't latched to the breast effectively during the first couple of feeds after birth, this can cause nipple damage, resulting in pain later on, even when the latch has been corrected. As the baby feeds frequently, the nipples aren't getting much time to heal in between, resulting in several days or even weeks of discomfort. Applying nipple cream before and after each feed, as well as ensuring the baby has a good latch, can help prevent sore nipples and aid the healing process. This is something a midwife or lactation consultant can support you with.

There are times when someone plans to breastfeed, but they are unable to for reasons such as insufficient glandular tissue (IGT), when there isn't enough milk-producing tissue in the breast. This affects approximately 5 per cent of new mothers. If a baby has persistent latch issues or conditions such as a cleft lip and palate, or the mum is feeding multiples and does not have enough milk for all babies (note that many twin mums are able to exclusively breastfeed their babies, as the breasts work on a supply-and-demand basis), other methods of feeding the baby might be needed. This could come in the form of expressing breastmilk and feeding via a bottle, donated breastmilk from a donor milk bank or formula feeding. If a mother and baby are separated briefly after birth for any reason or the mum is too unwell to breastfeed initially, the

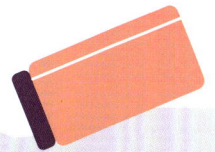

baby can be given donor or formula milk via a cup, bottle or syringe until breastfeeding can commence. Premature and sick babies in the NICU that are unable to suckle and feed may be given expressed milk via a nasogastric tube (NGT), until they are well and developed enough to learn how to feed directly from the breast.

For many women, breastfeeding is a wonderful, rewarding experience, which continues for many months or a few years. For others, the journey isn't so joyous, and they make the difficult decision to stop sooner than they had hoped. This can bring about feelings of disappointment, guilt and inadequacy. Any amount of breastfeeding is beneficial to babies, whether it is three weeks or three years, and what your baby needs most is a mum who is physically and emotionally well.

Some people do not want to breastfeed. They will have their own reasons for this and their wishes should be respected. It may be due to a previous traumatic breastfeeding experience, being from a family where breastfeeding is not the norm or never having been around people who breastfeed, pressure from a partner or family members who want to feed the baby, or historic sexual abuse. Some women simply don't like the thought of it, and if that's you, that is okay!

If you want to breastfeed but are facing pressure from family or a partner not to, it can be a very difficult situation to be in. Talking to your midwife about it may help as they can chat with you and your partner, and talk about any concerns they have, dispelling any myths in the process. Some mums who want their baby to have the benefits of breastmilk but do not wish to feed directly from the breast will express with a pump, and give it to them in a bottle instead.

FORMULA FEEDING

If you decide to formula feed from the beginning, you'll want to make sure you have everything you need ready before the birth. This includes enough formula and bottles, a steriliser and bottle-/teet-cleaning brushes. Powdered formula should be mixed with water that has been boiled, and fed to the baby within two hours of preparation. If it's not used straight away, it can be stored for 24 hours in a fridge, and warmed in a bottle warmer or a bowl of warm water. It must be used within two hours of coming out of the fridge. Most infant formulas are cow-protein based, and all bottles and teats need to be washed of all traces of milk before being sterilised to prevent bacteria growth. Pre-made cartons of formula are available but these are more expensive. They are handy, however, for taking into hospital when you give birth. Newborns should only drink stage-one formulas. 'Hungrier baby' milks are not scientifically proven to settle babies better – these milks are marketed at those hoping to get their baby to sleep for longer, but this often doesn't work. These milks contain more casein protein than whey, and casein is harder for babies to digest, often resulting in constipation.

Contrary to popular belief, formula-fed babies will still need to be fed throughout the night. All babies, whether breast or formula fed, have a biological need to feed often and that includes at night. Their stomachs are small, meaning they can only tolerate small amounts at a time. As the weeks and months go by, babies naturally start to sleep for longer, meaning more rest for you! To begin with, breastfed babies can feed anywhere between eight and twelve times or more per day, and formula-fed babies around eight to twelve times.

Paced bottle feeding is a method that can be used to prevent a baby drinking too quickly and developing too much air in the stomach, which can cause discomfort. You can do this when feeding expressed breastmilk or formula from a bottle. It involves using a slow-flow bottle teet and holding the baby in a semi-sitting position. The bottle should be in a horizontal position so that the teet is only half filled with milk. After the baby has had around five continuous sucks and swallows, tip the bottle down to allow the baby to have a break for a few seconds. Repeat until the baby has had enough. Signs of being full include no longer sucking after the break, turning away or pushing away from the teet. Don't be tempted to insist that the baby finishes every drop, as this may result in vomiting and belly ache.

COMBINATION FEEDING

Some parents like to both breastfeed and formula feed. This is called combination or combi feeding. I've worked with parents who have chosen to do this if they've had problems with exclusive breastfeeding, or those who feel that doing both will fit in better with daily routines such as work and other children. The ratio of feeding varies; it could be that every other feed is formula and breast, or mostly breast during the day and a couple of formula bottles at night.

There is no right or wrong way to combi feed, although I would advise establishing breastfeeding first in the early weeks before introducing a bottle if you plan to do so.

Feeding your baby is the perfect way to bond with them. If you bottle feed, hold them close while you feed them. Looking into their eyes, stroking, singing or talking to your baby are all ways to increase the maternal/parental bond between you and your little one.

ALCOHOL CONSUMPTION WHEN BREASTFEEDING

Drinking alcohol when breastfeeding doesn't pose the same risks as drinking when pregnant, but it's still not a good idea to consume large amounts at any given time. Regularly drinking large quantities and/or binge drinking can reduce your milk supply and may affect the baby. Traces of alcohol do enter breastmilk, but when consuming small amounts (1 to 2 units at any one time), it is unlikely to cause harm to the baby. The NHS recommends drinking no

more than 14 units of alcohol spread out throughout the week when breastfeeding to minimise any potential risks to your baby. The bigger issue of drinking vast amounts of alcohol when you have a newborn is your ability to care for them properly. If you are intoxicated, you should not care for your baby alone, and shouldn't bed-share with them.

If you drink alcohol, the odd glass of wine is unlikely to cause an issue, particularly if you allow a couple of hours to pass afterwards before feeding your baby.

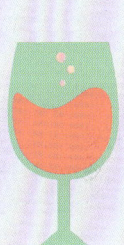
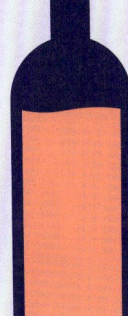

BOOBS, PUMPS AND BIG FEELINGS

I was very lucky that I wanted and was able to breastfeed with relative ease, so I chose to breastfeed each baby for the first four months of their life. My overriding memory of starting that journey is that when your milk comes in it is very emotional. So, as Marley says above, the colostrum gets produced initially, and then, on day three or four

after you give birth, you will start producing milk and your boobs will get extremely uncomfortable and feel very tight. And actually, without fail, when my boobs got enormous and incredibly sore, I always cried for a whole day for absolutely no reason. It was really emotional. And it felt dramatic – I thought there must be something wrong with me, but there wasn't; it was just that my milk had come in.

As somebody who went back to work at around four or five months postpartum, expressing and pumping became a big feature of my life. You can get electric or hand pumps and I tried both, but I felt that the electric ones were noisy and they can make you feel quite self-conscious if you're in a public place or a toilet cubicle at work trying to express milk. The hand pumps are silent – or at least almost silent – and they're very easy to use. I had more success expressing milk using a hand pump, so that's what I'd recommend, but what you choose will be dependent on your circumstances and preferences.

My worry with breastfeeding was that I was constantly thinking, *Is the baby getting enough milk? Am I producing enough milk?* That can be very stressful. But try not to worry about it; your body is an amazing machine, and it knows how much milk your baby needs. And if your baby isn't getting enough milk, it will feed for a little bit longer. You'll be thinking, *Oh my God, they're trying to get more milk out.* But actually,

they're trying to trigger the production of more milk, because when your baby sucks a little longer, your breasts produce more milk, so at the next feed the baby will have more milk to drink. The bigger your baby gets, the more it sucks, the more milk your breasts produce and the more the baby receives. The science behind it is incredible. But to help put your mind at rest, you can also keep an eye on your baby's nappies as they should be producing wet ones regularly. As Marley has outlined on page 237, your midwife will also have an eye on their weight and be checking their nappies.

Those early days are when I think you definitely want a pump nearby just to relieve your boobs a little, because the swelling and feeling of holding lots of milk in them is very intense. Sometimes I used to have to wake up in the night to relieve my boobs with a little bit of pumping, so make sure you've got everything you need to do that before you go to bed, so you're not having to walk around the house and really wake yourself up to get prepped to express.

The science behind it is incredible.

Your body is an amazing machine, and it knows how much milk your baby needs.

NAPPIES AND CLEANING

Changing a nappy is a quite a weird thing the first time you do it. Your baby's first poo can be quite disarming if you're not sure what to expect. The first poo is called meconium, and it is very dark and thick – a dark green or black, and hardly smells at all. It's what was formed in the baby's bowel during pregnancy and it takes a few days for this to pass, then, once they're feeding, the colour and consistency of their poo changes, to green around day two or three, then to brown/orange on day four or five, and yellow on day five or six.

For the first few days you'll only be changing a nappy a few times, but after the first week that escalates – fast! – and it can be up to twelve times over the course of a day and night. The type of nappy you opt for – whether disposable or reusable – will be up to you and your lifestyle. Since I had my babies, the reusable-nappy market has totally transformed and there are loads of brilliant options with pants and liners that are making it much easier to go down this route, which is kinder for the baby's skin, too. There is also an amazing array of biodegradable, zero-plastic baby wipes and so, if those are affordable to you, I would gently urge you to use those and do what you can to help with the environment, given how many nappies a baby will get through in the first two years of its life. There are also things like biodegradable nappy bags, and ways to buy things in bundles, but your choice has got to work for you, your baby and your lifestyle.

What is quite nice is that at this early stage, when babies are just drinking milk, the poo doesn't really smell, especially if you're breastfeeding. But let me tell you – it travels! And that means cleaning can become quite a mission. Just remember that your baby's bottom area is very sensitive, so be gentle. I was very worried, cleaning a girl's vagina, about poo getting in there and causing some kind of infection. But actually, all you have to do is get a baby wipe, and give the area a careful clean with that. If it is a wee you can just give it a wipe down. Most of the baby wipes available nowadays are very, very gentle as well as biodegradable. If it is a very messy poo, and it has gone inside, you can gently part your daughter's genitals and just give them a careful but thorough wipe from front to back. Don't ever go back to front because that can lead to infection, which is also why you want to try to keep the urethra clean. But you don't need to get overanxious about it. Very, very quickly it just becomes a natural part of cleaning your baby daughter and won't feel frightening or intimidating at all.

With a boy, it's much easier to give them a good clean. Just make sure you fold your son's penis to one side as you're cleaning it, because often they pee when they've got their nappy off, as they love the air. With a boy, the head of the penis will self-clean to some extent, so don't try to pull back the foreskin to clean it because it will still be attached to his penis and might tear. Also don't worry about swollen testicles. That is quite normal during the first few days – they can look really bright red and very swollen. It's completely harmless and quite common; it just means that fluid has collected there, and the swelling goes down in a few months. But if your baby's testicles are still swollen after a few months, do talk to your GP about it.

Bathtime is a good moment to just make sure the penis is nice and clean, as well as all the little creases in the nooks and crannies all around, but as I said, don't try to pull back the foreskin. The same goes for a girl – a bath is always a good time to make sure everything is properly clean.

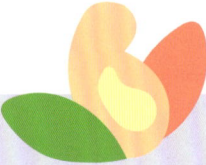

CLEANING THE UMBILICAL CORD

Midwife Marley

After the umbilical cord is clamped and cut, the remaining tissue, known as the umbilical stump, starts to turn black. Eventually it will harden and fall off on its own. You'll probably notice it in the nappy or your baby's clothing after a change. This process can take two weeks but usually happens after a week. You don't need to treat it with any special lotions or powders, just keep the area clean and dry. If you notice that the area around the cord stump is dirty – for example, from poo after a nappy change – gently wipe with cotton wool and warm water. Keep the nappy over the top of the cord or rolled down underneath it. Some nappies are shaped to allow the stump to dry out so it's not covered. This will also prevent friction and irritation to the area.

As the stump dries out, you may notice it starting to look a little sticky at the base. This is called 'sloughing' and is a normal part of the healing process. The stickiness soon dries out and turns darker in colour. If your baby's skin looks red and sore around the outside, is bleeding, oozing pus or swollen, and/or your baby has a temperature, seek advice from the maternity unit as this may be a sign of infection.

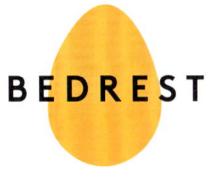

BEDREST

Getting some proper rest in the first few days after giving birth is really important because you are going to be shattered. You might have been in labour for many, many hours. After my first birth, when everybody had gone home, all the excitement was over, and it was just me and the baby, I was like, 'What do I do? I don't know what I'm doing. Help!' And what you should do is try to take it really, really easy for at least the first 24 to 48 hours. In fact, I recommend at least ten days' bedrest if that is possible, as this is what my midwife Caroline advised me to do. When I was pregnant with Holly she said, 'I advise everybody to have ten days' bedrest after they've had a baby.' I was really surprised by this because it felt so old-fashioned, and such a weird thing to do because at that time, it felt as though there was a certain pride in being able to get up and about with your baby and show him or her off within a few days. But Caroline said, 'When are you ever going to get an opportunity to spend this time with your newborn again? This is a once-in-a-lifetime opportunity.' Think about the physiological changes that your body's gone through – your uterus is shrinking back down, your whole vagina might be regrouping after what has been a pretty traumatic experience – so you just need give it some time to recuperate, heal and recover.

So, I did follow Caroline's advice and just rested as much as I could. She said bedrest but really you can go and rest on the sofa; there's just no need to get dressed. Do not be in a hurry to get out and do things. If I'm honest, I think I lasted till about day eight or nine, but I stayed in my pyjamas and I do remember those first days as some of the happiest I'd ever had. I stepped off the merry-go-round of life and just took time to experience the babies, feeding them, looking at them, talking to them, smiling at them and smelling them, and just forging all those memories. It was a really precious time. Of course, ten days at home isn't realistic for everyone, particularly if you have other children and there are nursery runs or school pick-ups and supermarket trips to be done. With other children around it's definitely harder to shut yourself off from the world, and you have to let them be part of those ten days. I remember Holly enjoyed the responsibilities of me asking her to help with certain things; it made her feel involved. But I would urge you to try to rest and savour as much time with your baby for as long as is possible for you.

Caroline had such a profound effect on my births, how I understood the whole process of having a baby and my recovery that I wanted to give her the opportunity to explain in her own words why she believes in the power of resting as much as you can. I know it's not feasible for everyone, but I find the theory behind it fascinating.

A NEW WORLD

Caroline Flint RN RM ADM, Midwife

Having a baby is like emigrating to a foreign country where you don't speak the language and don't understand the customs, all while feeling physically battered and emotionally exhausted. On top of that, no one else seems to understand what you are going through. It's an enormous transition.

First, it takes at least a year to fully recover physically from giving birth. Your body has been bombarded with hormones; every part of you has been stretched and bent; you may have surgical scars from a caesarean section or episiotomy. You have retained fluids so you are swollen and puffy and you are likely having to learn how to breastfeed a baby who is often reluctant and clueless as to what they should be doing – all they do is cry!

So, number one: you need time to recover, regroup and find your new place in the world; you need to rest and recuperate. You also need time to get to know your baby. So, I strongly suggest a 'babymoon' – 10 to 14 days in bed with minimal clothing on, next to a baby with minimal clothing on, and no visitors. You

will, however, need someone there to look after you, to tidy your bed, to cook your lunch/breakfast/dinner, to run the household, do the laundry, organise the shopping and run you a bath.

Your job is to get to know your baby. Get to know what they are saying to you, get to know their smell, get to know every nook and cranny of their face, how their skin feels and looks, how they always give a little signal before they poo. You may get bored, and that's fine; gentle music is soothing and lifts the spirits.

You are lying in bed and you are in the privacy of your bedroom. If you have other children, they will be able to come and spend time with you. They can have stories and sing with you, but basically you will be quite boring for them as you won't be doing much. Your body will begin to recover. You will need to pee frequently to get rid of the accumulation of fluid, and you will need to get up to change the baby's nappy. There is no danger of deep vein thrombosis if you are getting up and moving about often during the 24 hours of each day, always returning to your bed. You will doze and begin to recover from labour. Your tissues will begin to heal.

In order to promote healing, keep your perineum clean. If you have a bath, herbs boiled up in water and poured into the tub, such as calendula, St John's wort, lavender, rosemary and yarrow, can all feel very soothing and aid healing. When you wash your perineal area, be brave and touch it to make sure you have removed all the blood clots and dried-on debris. Dry it well with a soft towel or kitchen roll.

If you have a shower, put your herbal soak in a bowl that you can fit your genital area into – it is an area that can heal quite quickly.

You are getting to know your baby, beginning to fall in love with them. You are healing and being refreshed. If someone can give you a gentle massage, that can be incredibly helpful, but most important of all, just detach from the world for as long as you can. The more you rest and become familiar with your baby and your new life, the sooner you will embrace your strange new role. Once you are up and about, continue to rest in your bed every day until the baby no longer wakes during the night, which may be a very long time! Welcome to motherhood – the most significant role of all.

I strongly suggest a 'babymoon' – 10 to 14 days in bed with minimal clothing on, next to a baby with minimal clothing on, and no visitors.

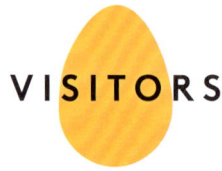

VISITORS

A really good piece of advice is not to have the world over to see your baby in the early days. It was such a huge temptation for me, particularly as an extrovert, to invite everybody I knew to meet my baby; with Holly especially, I wanted to show her off and I had loads of people over to visit all the time, yet looking back I feel it was a mistake, because what all your kind and well-meaning visitors will want to do is hold and cuddle the baby. But what you need them to do is help you with the cleaning and cooking because you want to hold and cuddle your baby. So I would suggest limiting the number you have round to one person a day, and getting those people to help you. Try not to have three or four people pop in – you're exhausted and it's just too much chat. And I know it's so often said, but it's true that when your baby's asleep, you need to try to use that time to get some sleep yourself, so the minute your baby goes down to bed, don't clean, don't wash, don't do anything. Lie down with your baby and go to sleep. At the end of the day, everyone is different, but I would just say think about it – because limiting visitors might allow you and your body the space you need to recover at your own pace, and to give your baby a gentle introduction to its new surroundings.

If friends ask what you want for the baby, say instead that you'd like vouchers for COOK meals (freezer meals made by hand – I'm not paid by them to say this!) as knowing you've got nutritious food ready to go is such a lifeline. Some of the useful tasks you could ask people to help with when they do come round are:

— giving the kitchen a clean

— unloading the dishwasher

— putting a wash on or hanging up the clothes from the machine

— bunging a meal from the freezer in the oven or whipping up a simple, nutritious meal for you for later

When I was doing my ten days' bedrest, I felt a lot of pressure from other people to be more active. They were saying things like, 'Aren't you going to get out of bed yet? Oh, you must be down because you're not going out. You need to get up and get outside.' If you are experiencing something similar, please do what you feel is right for you and set boundaries. It's really hard when you're feeling vulnerable and you've just had a baby to voice your opinion, but you need to practise lines that you think you would be able to deliver kindly but firmly. Things like, 'Thank you so much for your concern, but I know what I want to do.' If you always start with thanks, then the other person feels like they've done something good. For instance, 'Oh, that's really sweet, but actually, I'm really happy I'm going to do this.' Don't give them any room for manoeuvre.

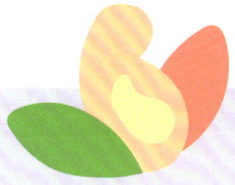

GOING OUT FOR THE FIRST TIME

Midwife Marley

Years ago, women were told to stay at home with their baby for weeks after the birth. As the years have gone on, life has made it harder for women to do this, particularly those with other children and little support. Twenty years ago, it was common for community midwives to carry out all postnatal visits within the parent(s)' home. Nowadays, increasing workloads often mean that some postnatal appointments are held in community settings like GP clinics, meaning that leaving the home tends to happen a lot earlier than it used to. For most new mums, going out for the first time after giving birth can be both exciting and daunting. It's normal to feel a mix of emotions – eagerness to escape the four walls of home, but also nervousness about leaving with a newborn in tow. The key is to plan ahead and be gentle with yourself as you navigate this new chapter. Here are some tips that might make your first outing smoother for both you and your baby:

— Your body has gone through a lot, and it's important to be mindful of your recovery. If you've had a vaginal birth, you might have stitches and still be experiencing tenderness or perineal discomfort.

— Walking short distances and sitting comfortably may take some time, so plan your trip accordingly. Some people are up and out of the house after four days; for others it could be 10 days or more – everyone is different. My suggestion would be to start by popping the baby in a pram and going for a short walk around the block or down the road, and seeing how you feel. Only do this if you are able to walk around the house without wincing with discomfort. If it's too uncomfortable to do so because of a caesarean or perineal stitches, rest for another couple of days before you try again.

— If you've had a caesarean section, take extra care with movement and lifting, and if possible, avoid going alone when you venture out for the first time.

— When you decide to go out for longer periods of time, be sure to take a few things with you for the journey, such as essentials like nappies, wipes, a change of clothes for your baby and feeding supplies (whether you're breastfeeding or bottle-feeding). Ensure you have drinks for yourself and any medication that you have been prescribed.

— Listen to your body. If you start feeling fatigued or overwhelmed during the outing, don't push yourself. It's okay to cut your trip short or ask for help from a partner or friend. Emotional recovery is just as important as physical recovery, so give yourself permission to take it slow.

The first outing is a learning experience. Each time will get easier, and before long, these trips will become part of your new routine. Take it one step at a time, and trust that you're doing great!

The first outing is a learning experience.

Each time will get easier, and before long, these trips will become part of your new routine.

Take it one step at a time, and trust that you're doing great!

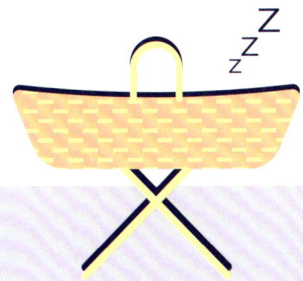

YOUR BABY'S SLEEP

Midwife Marley

Babies and sleep is probably one of the most searched-for topics on the internet for new parents. Because baby sleep patterns are so different to ours as adults, it can be really exhausting in the early days. I want to begin by saying that when your baby is born, they will have no concept of night or day as part of their sleep cycle (also known as the circadian rhythm), and it is not typical for a newborn to sleep for more than a few hours at a time. This applies throughout the day and night. Your baby will develop a sleeping pattern that resembles yours over time. It can be a long and exhausting time, but as the months go by, things usually get easier.

Newborns can sleep for up to 18 to 19 hours in any 24-hour period, broken into several sleep sessions lasting around one to three hours at any one time. The first 24 to 48 hours after birth, however, can be deceiving as newborns will generally sleep for longer stretches as they rest and

recover from being born. It's not unusual for a parent to say to me, 'They were sleeping for three to four hours the day they were born, and now they wake every 50 minutes!' It's important to know that babies need to feed regularly, which is part of the reason they wake so often. In the early days, if you are breastfeeding, the baby is consuming small quantities of colostrum, so it may feel like they are feeding constantly to encourage the 'full milk' to come in.

Like older children and adults, newborn sleep sessions are made up of light sleep, also known as rapid eye movement (REM), and deep sleep. During light sleep, the baby may wiggle around, make noises, grimace or open their eyes briefly. During deep sleep, they won't be as active, lying relatively still, and will be much quieter. Many parents ask about when to start a routine for their babies to help encourage them to sleep through the night. My advice would be to remember that tiny babies are not designed to sleep 10 to 12 hours straight at night. Bedtime routines are a great way to settle your baby and help them to learn the difference between night and day, but they will sleep through the night in their own time.

As a side note, the term 'sleeping through the night' in reference to babies means a six- or seven-hour stretch. A baby that goes to bed at 8 p.m., wakes at 11 p.m. or midnight for a feed, then sleeps until 6 or 7 a.m., would be classed as sleeping through. A simple bedtime routine may include a bath, feed, cuddle/story/lullaby/baby massage, before putting them down to sleep. Don't be alarmed if your baby starts to cry as soon as you put them down; it's not abnormal. Babies have a physiological need to be close to you. If you put them down when they are wide awake, they will probably fuss. Try putting them down to sleep gently and slowly when they are drowsy. Touch is one of the most powerful senses in babies so placing a hand on them if they become fussy lets them know you are still there.

SO WHEN DO BABIES START SLEEPING LONGER?

By around two to three months of age, they will have started developing a circadian rhythm but will still likely need to be fed during the night, albeit with longer sleep sessions.

By six months of age, babies are usually sleeping around 13 hours in a 24-hour period, which includes a couple of naps during the day of one or two hours. The majority of their sleep will be at night.

Babies can continue to have the odd daytime nap until two, three or even four years of age in some cases.

There are lots of variables that contribute to baby sleep cycles, including their age, sleeping environment, whether they have issues such as reflux or tongue tie, and their temperament. My five children slept through the night at vastly different ages – six months, nine months, two years, three years and eight years. They all had different needs, requiring different approaches to sleep. If you feel that your baby is waking excessively and you are finding it difficult to cope, contact your health visitor for support.

During the first six months of life, it's recommended by the WHO, NHS and safe sleep organisations such as the Lullaby Trust, that your baby sleeps in the same room as you. This applies to daytime naps, too. Research has shown that this reduces the risk of sudden infant death syndrome (SIDS). Your baby's sleeping space should be clear of heavy blankets, toys, teddy bears and cot bumpers. To keep baby warm at night when it's cold, a sleep bag is the safest option. These fasten around the shoulders, preventing the baby from wriggling down and covering their heads. With blankets, it's difficult to prevent this from happening. Baby sleeping bags have different thicknesses (referred to with a tog rating) depending on the environmental temperature. Be sure to check the guidance on the labels, which should tell you which tog to use.

Put your baby to sleep on their back, on a firm mattress. As they grow, they will learn to roll over and you may find that they adjust to their own preferred sleeping position. Pillows should not be placed in a cot until your baby is at least a year old. The room should be between 16 and 20°C (61 and 68°F), so you may want to get a thermometer for the room that your baby will be sleeping in.

CO-SLEEPING

Co-sleeping, also known as bed-sharing, is a controversial topic that causes division among parents. The safest place for a baby to sleep is in their own space, free of objects that can cause suffocation. Many parents, however, will choose to co-sleep to keep their baby settled. If you choose to co-sleep, here are some guidelines from the Lullaby Trust for doing it safely:

— Ensure your baby is well away from bedding such as pillows and duvets. Never cover your baby with an adult quilt.

— Do not allow pets or other children into the bed while the baby is there.

— Remove any slatted or decorated headboards and ensure there is no possibility of your baby becoming stuck in any gaps within the bedframe, particularly if the bed is against a wall.

— Do not fall asleep in an armchair or on a sofa with your baby.

Co-sleeping can be dangerous under the following circumstances and should be avoided:

— if any adults sleeping with the baby have consumed alcohol or drugs that induce sleepiness

— if anyone in the bed is a smoker or if the baby was exposed to smoking during pregnancy

— if the baby weighed less than 2.5kg (5½lb) at birth or was born prematurely before 37 weeks of pregnancy.

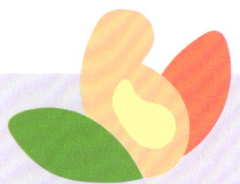

LIFE WITH TWINS AND MULTIPLES

Midwife Marley

If you've given birth to twins or multiples, the real fun begins when your babies come home. When you give birth to a singleton, it's much easier to follow their lead in terms of feeding. With two or more babies, it's not so easy, as you'll feel like you are constantly feeding and winding one baby or another. One of the best things I did when I had my twins was always to feed them together or one straight after the other. This prevented what I call 'mum's feed fatigue'. I also did things like bathing and trying to put them to sleep at the same time. Breastfeeding multiples is possible, but you may need support, so check out what local feeding support services are available before you give birth. If your babies are born premature, offering them breastmilk is recommended whether that is directly from the breast or via a pump/hand expressing. This is because preterm babies are more likely to suffer problems with their gut, and breastmilk can help protect them from this. If you reach 36 weeks of pregnancy, ask your midwife or infant feeding specialist for information on colostrum harvesting (see page 151). This can help you build up a little supply prior to the birth and may support your supply in the first few days after birth.

Support from those around you is essential after having one baby, let alone two or three! Check in with your family and friends and write a list of ways that they can be of help. This could be bringing you essential supplies like bread and milk, or watching the babies for five minutes so that you can take a shower.

If you've had identical babies, you may be worried that you'll get them confused. Over time you will identify differences such as head shape, birthmarks, leg length and personalities. In the early days a simple way to identify them is to dress them in different colours. You could also use a marker pen to draw a symbol on the front of their nappy each time you change them. You won't need to do this for long, though, as very quickly you'll spot differences that are super-obvious to you, even if they're not to others.

YOUR STORIES

'Twins!?!?! WTF?'— Kathryn

My pregnancy was already a bit of a surprise for myself and my partner. Then we had a scan at 11 weeks and the sonographer said, 'Do you see what I see?' Yes, there was another baby alongside the first one we saw. OH MY GOD! I must have said that about 209 times alongside other expletives. I had awful morning sickness – it was on the verge of being HG but it had a three-day cycle, which meant I could eat and drink fairly normally on one day a week so that kept me out of hospital. Being self-employed I would not be paid if I took time off. I stopped being sick around 29 weeks thankfully. The rest of my pregnancy was okay except that I was huge. My twins shared a placenta so I was kept a close eye on. There is a risk of twin-to-twin transfusion syndrome with twins that share a placenta, which means that one baby takes more of the nutrients away from the other. If it is severe it can lead to both babies dying. Thankfully there was no sign of this in my pregnancy and I comfortably got to 37 weeks and they talked about induction. I was ready to evacuate so agreed. Induction was a very long-winded process. I had a pessary Friday morning, spent the day walking, had another Friday evening, slept for a bit, by early Saturday morning I was dilated enough to break my waters. I then was told to mobilise again; we found the stairs and went up and down quite a bit. They then started me on the drip. Contractions came steadily. I got to the stage where I felt I needed an epidural as it was getting difficult to manage. I now know this can slow down labour and that's exactly what it did. They upped the dose of the drip, then the babies began to show signs of distress

so they suggested a C-section may be necessary. I agreed as I was struggling. We were prepped and whisked in almost immediately and my twins were born 1 minute apart to the sound of Stevie Wonder. One came out screaming, the other came out calmly looking around but breathing. This sums up their different personalities, even now. I couldn't believe how quickly they were born. It took a lot longer to sew me back together. We were taken to recovery and both babies latched separately and breastfed for several minutes each. This was the point I decided I just had to breastfeed. I was discharged and the next two weeks were quite challenging. I was in a lot of pain, couldn't move easily and breastfeeding two babies was a lot to deal with! My mum was amazing. She would cuddle, change, settle babies and I would feed them. I had a wonderful midwife who showed me how to tandem feed. This was the key!

Davina: Kathryn, I think lots of people have often wondered what it would feel like if they were told they were having twins, and I think it would be a feeling of great shock. But what's amazing is how you just got into the correct mindset, and that's so amazing. I love the fact that your mum was on hand to help and you had a fantastic midwife. Support is everything. And if you don't have a mum around, make sure you try and get friends to maybe come and help you at the beginning. Because I imagine until you get a system in place, those first few weeks are carnage. But, so many congratulations.

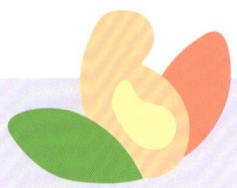

DIFFERENT CRIES AND SETTLING YOUR BABY

Midwife Marley

As a new parent, one of the most challenging tasks is learning to understand what your baby's cries mean. This can be overwhelming in the early days as you try to figure out why your baby is crying, particularly if things like feeding or holding them are not settling them down. With time, however, you'll begin to notice that different cries can mean different things, and you'll develop an understanding of these signals so that you can meet your baby's needs.

WHY DO BABIES CRY?

Newborns cry for many reasons, but most of the time it's because they need something. Babies cannot talk, so crying is their natural way of signalling hunger, discomfort, tiredness, or simply the need for comfort and closeness. It's important to remember that babies do not cry for the sake of it, although sometimes, it really can feel like it. Newborns also do not cry with tears for the first month or so, which leads some people to believe that the crying is not genuine. Crying often peaks between six and eight weeks of age and usually begins to settle by the time they are three to four months old.

A baby's cry could be mean a number of things, including:

— **Hunger:** This is one of the most common reasons a baby cries. A hungry cry is usually rhythmic and repetitive, and usually follows feeding cues such as sucking on their hands, rooting (turning their head towards anything that touches their cheek), wriggling or smacking their lips. These signs can happen for several minutes before crying begins. The crying will escalate quickly.

— **Discomfort:** Whether it's a dirty nappy, too tight clothing, being too hot or cold, or being in a position they don't like, discomfort can cause a cry. This cry may sound fussy or whiny. Checking for common physical discomforts like a wet nappy, the temperature or clothing tightness can help. Check your baby's fingers, toes and baby boys' genitals often, as sometimes adult hair can get wrapped tightly around them, causing pain and restricting blood flow. Postpartum hair loss is a common culprit for this.

— **Tiredness:** An overtired baby often becomes irritable and harder to soothe. The cry may start softly but can escalate quickly if they're struggling to fall asleep. You may also notice older babies rubbing their eyes or scratching their heads when tired. As a baby grows, you will begin to notice their sleep patterns. When you know your baby is due for a nap, make sure the environment is conducive to this, i.e. low lights, blackout blinds if possible and minimal noise.

— **Gas or colic:** If your baby is crying intensely and arching their back, they may be experiencing gas or colic (see box below). This cry can be high-pitched and accompanied by physical tension. Gentle belly rubs or bicycle leg movements can sometimes help relieve the discomfort.

— **Overstimulation:** Sometimes, babies cry when there's too much going on around them – bright lights, loud noises or too many people. This type of cry may sound like fussing or frustration.

— **Loneliness:** Babies also cry because they need comfort or want to be held. This is often a softer, more insistent cry. In the first few months of life, they are still adjusting to life outside the womb, so it isn't uncommon for them to want to be near you.

HOW TO SETTLE YOUR BABY

The way each baby is settled will vary greatly. If all obvious needs have been met (i.e. feeding, winding, changing, etc.), there are several techniques you can use. The Seven Ss is a great place to start:

1. Swaddle

Swaddling refers to wrapping a baby snugly in a thin wrap, keeping their arms down but allowing some movement for their hips and legs. This recreates the snugness of the womb and helps the baby feel secure. Not all babies like to be swaddled, but many will settle and enjoy the security. The Lullaby Trust has some important safety tips when doing this:

— Only use a lightweight wrap or sheet.

— Ensure they are not over-clothed when swaddling so that they don't overheat.

— Always place them on their back when swaddled and ensure their head is uncovered when indoors.

— Ensure they are swaddled securely around the shoulders – not the neck – and loosely around the hips. The legs should not be bound straight; they should be able to flex them into a 'frog' position.

You should **not** swaddle a baby when they are able to roll onto their side by themselves, when they have a fever or are unwell, or if they are sharing a bed with you. More information and infographics on swaddling can be found here: https://www.lullabytrust.org.uk/safer-sleep-advice/product-information/swaddling-slings/

2. Side or stomach position

Hold the baby on their side or stomach while soothing (but always place them on their back to sleep). This position helps reduce the Moro (startle) reflex and can help calm the baby. It can also help with the release of air bubbles in the digestive tract.

3. Shushing

Make a 'shhhh' sound close to the baby's ear. This mimics the whooshing noises they heard in the womb and can help block out other sounds that may be disturbing them. You can try this while rocking them side to side over your shoulder and lightly patting their back.

4. Swing

Babies love motion! For many people, rocking side to side when a baby is in their arms is instinctive. Gently rock or sway the baby back and forth, either in your arms or in a baby swing. Rhythmic movement mimics the motion experienced in the womb and can calm a fussy baby.

5. Suck

Offer a pacifier, clean finger or breast to help the baby suck. Sucking is naturally soothing and helps regulate the baby's heartbeat and breathing. Many babies will immediately calm down and drift off while being comforted through sucking.

6. Sling

Carrying the baby in a sling or carrier, also known as babywearing, is a popular way to calm them when they're crying and unsettled. If you are moving around, the motion will offer comfort, along with your warmth and the sound of your heartbeat. They will also have the security of being close to you while you remain hands-free to carry out other tasks should you need to. The Consortium of UK Sling Manufacturers and Retailers offers guidance in the form of the acronym TICKS, to help keep your baby safe and close in a sling:

— **T**ight

— **I**n view at all times

— **C**lose enough to kiss

— **K**eep chin off the chest

— **S**upported back

The full guidance can be found here: https://babyslingsafety.co.uk/ticks.pdf

7. Skin-to-skin

Skin-to-skin contact (see page 217) isn't only beneficial at birth. Parents can soothe and bond with their babies through skin-to-skin at any time. It helps your baby's body to self-regulate, helping their heart rate, temperature and breathing to stabilise. This in turn can their lower stress hormones when crying, providing comfort to your baby.

WHAT IS COLIC?

You may have heard of the term 'colic' without really knowing what it means. In adults it is often used to refer to gripey abdominal pains that accompany an upset stomach. In babies, this term becomes confusing because the definition officially refers to a baby that cries for long periods of time with no obvious cause. It is a sign that the baby is experiencing discomfort somewhere, usually the abdomen, but not actually a diagnosis.

If your baby cries for more than three hours per day, at least three times a week for more than a couple of weeks, it may be classed as colic. No one is sure what causes colic in babies, but it is thought that digestive issues may contribute to it. This could be a build-up of air bubbles in the stomach from feeding, causing trapped wind, or a premature digestive system, or even sensitivity to cow's protein in formula milk.

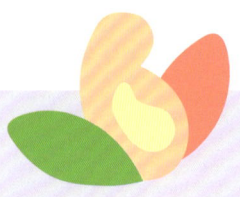

IDENTIFYING IF SOMETHING IS WRONG WITH YOUR NEWBORN BABY

Midwife Marley

As a new parent, it's natural to worry about your baby's health, especially when they can't tell you how they feel. Sometimes it can feel like we are questioning every new sound or movement they make, wondering if it could mean that something is wrong. Being on high alert is a natural response to having the responsibility of caring for a new baby. While most newborns experience a range of normal behaviours and minor discomforts, there are some signs that may indicate that something is wrong. Recognising these early can help you respond quickly and get medical advice when needed.

UNUSUAL CRYING

Crying is your baby's main way of communicating, but if your newborn's cry seems suddenly different – more high-pitched, unusually weak or constant – it could signal distress. Persistent, inconsolable crying, especially if accompanied by other symptoms like fever or changes in behaviour, might require medical attention.

CHANGES IN FEEDING OR WEIGHT GAIN

Newborns typically feed at least 8 to 12 times in a 24-hour period, whether breastfed or bottle-fed. If your baby suddenly stops feeding well, refuses to eat or vomits frequently, it may be a sign that they are unwell. Poor feeding can lead to dehydration, which needs urgent treatment. If your baby is not gaining weight or appears to lose weight, contact your healthcare provider.

DIFFICULTY BREATHING

It's normal for newborn babies to breathe fast at around 40–60 breaths per minute. If you notice your baby is breathing much faster than this, is grunting or seems to struggle for breath (nostrils flaring, chest retracting with each breath), this could be a sign of respiratory distress. In this case, seek immediate medical attention.

FEVER OR LETHARGY

A fever of 38°C (100.4°F) or higher in a newborn is cause for concern and should be checked by a doctor immediately. A digital thermometer placed in the crook of your baby's armpit with their arm down by their side will give you an accurate reading if you suspect that they feel too hot. Babies do sleep a lot, but if they suddenly develop extreme sleepiness, have trouble waking or difficulty staying awake for feedings, this should also be checked out.

SKIN COLOUR CHANGES

Keep an eye on your baby's skin. Bluish lips, a pale complexion or severe yellowing (jaundice) may indicate an underlying issue. Mild jaundice is common in the early days and usually resolves by itself with plenty of feeding. If in doubt, contact your midwife for advice. Lots of babies develop rashes at around four to six weeks of age, which usually clear within a couple of weeks. This is thought to be caused by the adjustment to their new environment. If your baby develops a purple/deep-red rash that is flat and doesn't disappear when pressed with a glass tumbler, this could be a sign of a serious infection called meningitis, particularly if accompanied with a fever and floppiness. If your baby presents with this rash, call 999 for an urgent assessment.

Always trust your instincts. If something feels off, it's always better to seek medical advice early.

Don't ever worry about wasting anyone's time; it's best to be safe and get your baby checked out.

DON'T BE AFRAID TO ASK FOR HELP

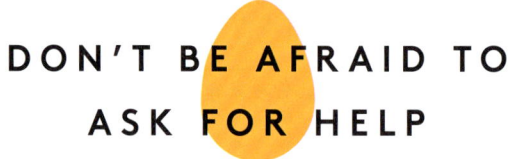

As women, we can excel at 'putting a brave face on', being stoic and strong, and coping with challenges alone – and this is particularly common after giving birth.

There is this all-too-pervasive belief or expectation that when motherhood arrives we should automatically know what we are doing, be in command of this situation and thrive – that life with our new baby is blissful, and feeling anything other than overwhelming joy and contentment in this new phase of our life is abnormal or shameful.

But I really, really want to dispel that assumption. Of course, life with a baby CAN be blissful and life-changing in magical ways, but it is also hard and scary, and there are lots of things that can make us anxious, so it's a time when we really shouldn't be putting a brave face on things at all – we need to be asking for help and support. And we need to be very mindful of our own health and wellbeing, asking ourselves how we're feeling and acknowledging when we're not feeling okay – or feeling low.

Having disrupted sleep and feeling very, very tired can also amplify all these feelings and fears, making the risk of our mental health spiralling downwards even greater. Birth can create a huge emotional upheaval as well as a physical one, and we need support to navigate all that arises from that change. The reality is that many of us will feel bouts of the 'blues', and as Marley outlines on page 276, 1 in 10 women will experience a mental-health condition that is much more serious than this – postnatal depression needs rapid attention and treatment because it puts lives at risk. So, if any of the following feelings or thoughts resonate with you, please, please seek help. We've added places to turn to at the back of the book (see page 311).

The reality is that many of us will feel bouts of the 'blues' and 1 in 10 women will experience postnatal depression.

YOUR STORIES

'No one really prepares you for how much you disappear after the baby arrives. Everyone tells you about the sleepless nights, the feeding, the nappies. But no one says, *you might wake up one day and not recognise yourself at all.*' — Cathy

I remember staring at the clothes in my wardrobe and thinking, who even wore these? I didn't know what suited me anymore. My body felt unfamiliar, my moods were unpredictable, I cried at anything and I couldn't remember the last time I'd felt like a person with her own wants and plans – not just a vessel for feeding, soothing, surviving. I didn't do anything of the things I used to love doing.

I tried to hold on to myself in small ways: putting on mascara even if I wasn't going anywhere, reading a book while the baby napped (if they napped), going for short walks alone just to hear my own footsteps, or checking in with friends without talking about babies. But even then, I felt like I was pretending. Like I was play-acting the role of 'normal' while feeling anything but.

It was destabilising – how much love I had for this tiny human, and how little love I seemed to have left for myself.

Slowly, I'm finding my way through, but I do feel like I've lost some bit of myself that has gone forever.

Davina: Thanks for your story, Cathy. It is funny how it's almost a crime to say if you're finding it difficult, but I think all of us do at some point; it is such a lot to contend with. And I think that being honest and talking about it really helps. So well done and well done for all the ways that you have tried to counter these feelings. They were very helpful to read.

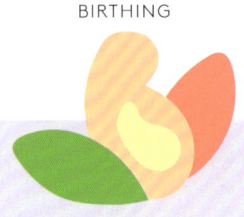

EMOTIONS AND POSTNATAL DEPRESSION

Midwife Marley

Over 80 per cent of women will go through some kind of emotional transition after having a baby. For the vast majority, this manifests itself in the form of what we call the 'baby blues'.

It's common to feel emotional and weepy a few days after giving birth, particularly if you've had a difficult birth or are worn out from lack of sleep while attempting to heal. Most women find that after a few days, their mood improves as they start to heal and settle into life with a new baby.

Postnatal depression is more serious than the 'baby blues' and affects around 1 in 10 people after birth. If the initial weepiness develops into low mood and persists for a more than a couple of weeks, it could be postnatal depression. There are many other signs of postnatal depression, including:

— persistent sadness and low mood

— loss of interest in activities you used to find pleasurable

— having difficulty in bonding with your baby

— lack of energy

— insomnia

— feelings of guilt or hopelessness

— problems concentrating

Postnatal depression can affect anyone, regardless of whether they have previously suffered with mental health concerns or not. Midwives, health visitors and GPs are all there to help and offer support – the first step is to talk to someone.

Postnatal anxiety is often reported after birth, too, and can be mistaken for depression. Postnatal anxiety comes with some of the symptoms of depression, but without the sadness. It is associated more with excessive worrying and intrusive thoughts that many would consider to be irrational.

The least common form of mental illness after birth is postpartum psychosis, which affects around 1 in 1,000 new mothers. It begins very rapidly, within the first couple of weeks of birth, and is a medical emergency. Signs and symptoms include:

— hallucinations (seeing, smelling or hearing things that aren't really there)

— mania (bouts of feeling overly energetic or 'high'; for example, racing thoughts and speech, or a complete loss of inhibitions)

— delusions (believing things that are not true)

— depression (symptoms of depression in addition to the other symptoms listed)

— confusion (the inability to make sense of surroundings, or forgetting names, places, etc).

Postpartum psychosis can be extremely scary for anyone experiencing it, as well as for family and friends. Treatment and recovery come with early diagnosis, although it can be a long road.

It's important to talk to someone if you're experiencing any of the symptoms of postnatal depression, anxiety or psychosis. Suffering with a postnatal mental illness does not make anyone a bad parent, nor does it mean they do not love their baby. They are illnesses that need to be treated as such.

Family and partners can reach out to health professionals if they are concerned about a loved one.

Postpartum depression and anxiety are prevalent, but can usually be treated effectively. It may take some time for women to recover, so please just acknowledge that it's a case of being patient and following the treatment programme recommended.

I want to emphasise that the first week of having a baby can be really overwhelming for women. You have a massive surge of hormones on the day you give birth, and they will still be in your body for a few days, then you get a bit of a crash. As I said, with my first, I cried non-stop when my milk came in on the fourth day. But as Marley explained, postnatal depression is very different to the 'baby blues' and doesn't go away on its own, so please seek support. And if you're a partner or friend reading this, please step in if you feel you need to.

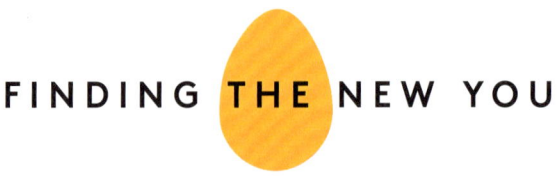

FINDING THE NEW YOU

One of the other elements of motherhood that has rarely been discussed openly and widely until the last few years is the transition and identity shift that comes with suddenly becoming a mother. So much is written and spoken about the birth itself, but we've tended to focus less on the huge psychological, emotional and physical changes a woman experiences and how they affect her and her sense of identity.

For most women, becoming a mother means that you have to figure out and define a whole new identity for yourself, and this can feel incredibly daunting, frightening and at times overwhelming.

Happily, as a society we're finally beginning to recognise this transition more formally, and the concept of 'matrescence' has been acknowledged and identified as a stage that women need support with.

I have always loved my career and prided myself in the fact that I am unashamedly ambitious. I want to do well. I want to succeed. I loved working, but I remember the shock of giving birth to Holly and looking at her and asking myself, *How will I ever work again? How will I ever enjoy working again? And will I ever be able to work without feeling really guilty about leaving her?*, and I found that really difficult to navigate.

So I'm really delighted to have clinical psychologist Dr Caroline Boyd talk about navigating matrescence and outline the support available to women.

Caroline has over 10 years' experience working in the NHS and mental-health settings, and she supports parents from pregnancy to childbirth and beyond.

Becoming a mother means that you have to figure out and define a whole new identity for yourself.

MATRESCENCE

Dr Caroline Boyd, Perinatal Clinical Psychologist and Author

Becoming a mother blasts us wide open. We can feel all at sea as we grapple with our new identity amid the huge responsibility of caring for a tiny person. This identity transition has been called 'matrescence' – it compares the process of becoming a mother to the huge changes that arise in adolescence. Just as teenagers navigate emotionally turbulent waters, so too do new mums, through significant brain, body and relationship changes. The term matrescence, coined in 1973 by anthropologist Dana Raphael, offers a map for the messy, mind-bending, heart-opening process of 'mother-becoming'. Unlike traditional models, which have focused heavily on the child, matrescence places the mother at the heart.

Of course, each woman's experience of matrescence is personal – depending on her quality of support, cultural stories, childhood experiences (including trauma and adversity), difficulties conceiving, baby loss and experiences of feeling 'othered' (linked, for example, to race, class and sexuality). However, a central theme of matrescence focuses on the mother (or primary caregiver) truly taking care of her mind and body – for the sake of her sanity and self-esteem as well as her baby's wellbeing. Matrescence normalises and validates the intense emotions new mums feel – allowing women to exhale with relief knowing they're not alone. There are four important areas to consider as you move through matrescence. I highlight these below, along with the tools that can help you cope and empower you on your journey.

1   THE SOCIAL

We're not designed to raise our baby in isolation as we do in individualistic Western cultures, but rather in groups as our ancestors did. All new mothers need the help of 'alloparents' (allo means 'other'), be they family members, friends or paid helpers, allowing them to rest and heal, away from modern pressures to 'bounce back'. They also need help from someone more experienced to teach them those mothering skills, particularly those new mothers who weren't supported to feel safe, seen and soothed growing up. These skills aren't 'innate' to women as the myth of 'Supermum' would have us believe.

Ask for help: I strongly encourage women to ask for help – whether this is enlisting helpers for practical tasks such as washing and cooking, or accessing professional help for struggles, be they related to tensions in the partner relationship, birth injury or breastfeeding. Society's lack of structural support for mothers is a sign of systemic failure, not a personal one. I urge women to self-advocate in the healthcare system with the message that getting help isn't a sign of weakness or failure – rather it shows strength, courage and commitment to improving things for the whole family.

2   THE PSYCHOLOGICAL

In the early days of parenting, we can experience a complex kaleidoscope of emotions – sometimes in a single day. This is known as the emotional push–pull: feeling pushed towards caring for our baby but also pulled away to focus on our other identities, leaving us yearning for physical and emotional space. The conflict around wanting to meet the needs of our baby as well as our own can bring intense discomfort – after all, this is a job we're *supposed* to be enjoying. It's meant to be *instinctual*.

But with 93 per cent of mums saying they feel their identity has been reduced to just one – mother – it's no wonder we might long for the familiarity of pre-baby life or experience fleeting moments of regret during this tumultuous time.

Allow all your feelings: What can really help is naming these confusing, difficult feelings – to take a small risk and share how we're feeling with an empathetic friend or trusted professional can help us process and make sense of these emotions. It's important to allow ourselves to grieve the losses that come with early motherhood, which may include spontaneity, assured sleep and time alone, as well as honour the gains. This means learning to notice our own emotions with kindness – and without self-blame.

3   THE NEUROBIOLOGICAL

Exciting new evidence suggests that first-time mothers undergo long-lasting shifts in the brain during pregnancy.[52] Affected brain regions are associated with theory of mind, the ability to empathise and understand another's perspective. This neural rewiring is understood to be adaptive – preparing us to recognise our baby's needs, enhancing our ability to respond to our baby sensitively and to perceived threats. Evidence of these amazing maternal brain changes really normalises the intense desire many new mums feel – often experienced as anxiety – to protect their new baby. It can be reassuring to know that feelings of overwhelm, as we adjust to the sheer responsibility, are signs that our radically reshaped brain is doing just what it's designed to do.

Understand why scary, intrusive thoughts occur: However, feeling so at one with your baby can feel all-consuming at times, filling you with anxiety and urgency when, for example, they cry. You may feel so tired you fear your baby might inadvertently come to harm. These fears are taboo yet really common. We know nearly every single woman experiences scary, intrusive thoughts of harm befalling her child, such as word thoughts ('What if my baby stops breathing?') and vivid visions of dropping them. One in two women also report unwanted thoughts of intentionally harming their baby – even though they would never deliberately hurt their child. These are unlike the kinds of thoughts arising in postpartum psychosis, which can include mania, delusions and hallucinations; intrusive thoughts don't sit comfortably with women and tend to evoke intense shame, horror and guilt. The very fact mums feel ashamed or horrified about having these thoughts is a strong sign that they're not going to

hurt their baby. Of course, intention is key. If you find yourself having an overwhelming desire or intention to hurt yourself or your baby, please seek help urgently.

What can really help is to understand intrusive thoughts as an effective warning system – helping you adapt to the huge responsibility of having a tiny baby. Talk about your thoughts with someone supportive to help you feel validated and less alone. Interpreting these thoughts to mean you're 'bad' or 'mad', or that you might act on them, empowers them, making them harder to dismiss. Practise mindfulness skills to separate yourself from your thoughts. Acknowledge them with kindness and without judgment, then try to let them go. Tell yourself: 'They don't mean I am a bad person. I'm a good enough mum and I am safe.'

4   GOOD-ENOUGH MOTHERING

The 'Supermum' fairytale tells us that perfection in parenting is possible if only we try hard enough. Yet we know that, in reality, even the most attuned mothers only get it 'right' – tuning in and responding sensitively to meet their baby's needs – around a third of the time. Matrescence supports us to move towards self-acceptance as a 'good-enough' mother.

Learn to self-soothe: Many mums tell me they feel they're failing when they don't respond 'perfectly' to challenging newborn moments such as long bouts of crying and sleepless nights. Yet our baby's cry is designed to elicit a strong reaction – often our responses in these moments are shaped by our previous experiences and the way our nervous systems typically react to stress. What's most important is finding ways to cope when we feel triggered – for example, in response to our baby crying.

My Three Rs (Regulate, Reconnect and Repair) exercise helps us to acknowledge and soothe our big emotions and reconnect with our babies:

Regulate: Put your baby down safely, or hand them over to someone else. Splash your face with cold water. Focus on breathing in for three counts, and exhaling steadily for six counts.

Reconnect with yourself: Notice and name your feelings. For example: 'I'm feeling exhausted/stressed/angry/fed up.' Notice your inner critic: is it negatively comparing you to others or an idealised you? The antidote to shame is empathy. Tell yourself gently: 'It's okay to struggle – I'm human. These feelings will pass and I'll find a way through this. I am a good, loving mum.'

Repair: After self-soothing, repair with your baby. Cuddle them and help them understand their feelings. Say softly: 'Crying is your way of communicating – I hear you. It's okay, Mummy's here.' Then find ways to soothe your baby that also soothe you. This could be gently swaying together or listening to relaxing music.

Matrescence is a transformative, if at times painful, process. As we adjust, our 'mother-becoming' offers a unique opportunity for growth as we re-evaluate old stories and let go of patterns that no longer serve us. Through gently exploring our new identity, we can deepen our self-awareness and feel empowered to mother in a way that fits for us.

Matrescence normalises and validates the intense emotions new mums feel.

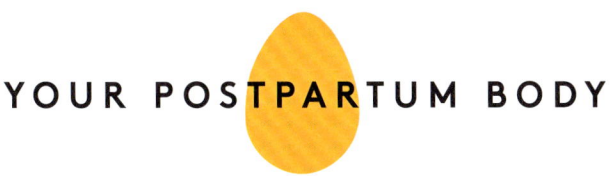

YOUR POSTPARTUM BODY

The statistics are shocking: according to the Mental Health Foundation, 41 per cent of women surveyed said they felt more negatively about their body image after pregnancy compared to before they were pregnant (23 per cent felt slightly more negative and 18 per cent much more negative). Only 12 per cent said they felt more positively about their body image post-pregnancy.[53]

In many ways, that's no surprise, as we are living in an age in which public discourse around 'postpartum bodies' and the need to transform and regain our 'pre-pregnancy bod' is rife; it is everywhere, intense and hard to ignore. However we feel about our shape, and regardless of how confident we are and whether we feel immense pride in what our body has just achieved, it's hard not to be impacted by all the messaging telling us to shed that 'pregnancy weight' as quickly as we can.

But this is my plea: I urge you to accept and respect the changes in your postpartum body. Because your body IS going to change. It's been through a massive physical transformation – stretched and pulled and expanded – to allow you to carry and grow your newborn, and it's just not designed to 'bounce back' from that experience. I ballooned over the course of each of my pregnancies, and there was no way my body was going to look like it had before the births in six months. I'd resigned myself to at least nine months up, nine

months down, and even though social media didn't exist when I was pregnant with Holly and Tilly, I was on *Big Brother*, and I literally played out my pregnancies on television and everybody could see how they ravaged my body. I was also fitness lady – I was Workout DVD girl – and I wasn't bouncing back.

So, you might be comparing yourself to other people and looking at all the gym-bunny bodies on Instagram on their postpartum journeys, but I really want to impress upon you not to look at those images and not to compare your body to theirs. You are you; you are unique – with your own individual genetics that will also play into how quickly you can 'snap back' – and you need to take things at your own pace as you find strength and allow your body to heal and recover from birth.

Childbirth is an incredible thing, so we need to learn to accept, be grateful for and inhabit our postpartum body, and remind ourselves that bodies aren't meant to reconfigure in a matter of weeks, or even months.

I know it won't be easy – there were days when I looked at myself in the mirror and just thought I looked exhausted and not like myself, but I found that the thing that made me feel better was just putting on a little bit of make-up. It wasn't for anybody else, it was just for me to feel like I'd made an effort by putting on a bit of mascara or some lip gloss. And it was about telling myself that I was worth making an effort for. Because when you've had a baby, it is very, very easy to forget to do things for yourself.

We must also remember that it isn't shameful or wrong not to love our bodies post-birth. We need to normalise those feelings and make women feel they can speak up and share their experiences and challenges. That honesty and candour helps us all understand that we're not alone and others are going through the same thing we are. And if you do find yourself feeling really demoralised by social media, perhaps take a break from it for a while. Just enjoy your time with your baby.

How you feel about your body may affect other areas of your life, including when you feel ready and able to start having sex again after birth.

I was grateful to the midwives and the doctor who said, 'Don't really think about it for six weeks. Let yourself heal and repair down there,' because it was nice for both me and my partner to know that it was not on the agenda. But some women may feel their desire for intimacy return quite quickly, and yet be nervous of penetrative sex, worried about how their partner is going to feel about their postpartum body, or experiencing other psychological barriers to being intimate again.

It can be quite a sensitive and complex issue, for both women and men, so we've asked Dr Karen Gurney – a wonderful clinical psychologist who specialises in helping couples and individuals overcome sexual problems – to dive into this and talk about some of the barriers and potential solutions to rekindling sexual activity with a partner when you're ready.

I was grateful to the midwives and the doctor who said,

'Don't really think about sex for six weeks. Let yourself heal and repair down there.'

SEX POSTPARTUM: ADDRESSING YOUR CONCERNS

Dr Karen Gurney, Consultant Clinical Psychologist

Sexual satisfaction declines in the first 12 months of being a parent for a third to half of all new parents.[54] Sexual difficulties, such as painful sex, or lack of arousal, desire and orgasm, are common for new parents, particularly in that first year. Around 90 per cent of parents report one or more sexual concerns, although these often resolve themselves by 12 months after birth.[55]

In the first six months to a year after having a new baby, sex often takes a back seat, and this is entirely normal. Just over half of new parents get back to penetrative sex in the first eight weeks and find this is fine for them;[56] by three months this figure has risen to 89 per cent.[57] Despite most couples trying penetrative sex in the first few months, the frequency of penetrative sex for most people doesn't go back to how things were pre-pregnancy until usually after the first year, and for many not for years.

The speed at which people return to having penetrative sex is (unsurprisingly) dependent on how their birth went. Those who had a vaginal birth without the use of instruments (such as forceps), episiotomy or a second-, third- or fourth-degree tear are more likely to resume sex earlier than those who didn't.[58]

Challenges with sex in the first year are due to a combination of factors, including the physical and psychological recovery after birth, sleep deprivation, the stress of having a new baby, the new increase in workload and loss of time, a change in body image, and sometimes the relationship challenges of becoming new parents. Studies tell us that having even one hour extra of sleep a night can increase our chances of having sex the next day by a whopping 14 per cent![59] We also know that sleeping poorly is associated with reduced sexual satisfaction and reduced frequency of sex. Basically, if you're not getting much sleep, don't expect to want much sex.[60]

The impact of sensory overload from breastfeeding, or being a primary caregiver more generally, along with the breasts feeling like an area with a changed meaning, sensitivity or appearance, can be enough to block any emerging sexual desire. The hormones that maintain the production of breastmilk can also prevent desire and make vaginal penetration more uncomfortable. This will resolve when breastfeeding stops. Crucially, if we can't communicate easily about this when we want to be sexual – for example, 'I want to leave my top on,' or, 'Please don't touch my breasts' – this can impact on our motivation to go there. Instead, we might reduce this discomfort by simply avoiding the whole thing rather than talking about what adjustments might make it doable.

Body image and sex do, of course, go hand in hand, especially when we are talking about intimate areas of our anatomy. Whether or not people have had tears, they can harbour fears that their vagina will be stretched to the point where they or their partner might not enjoy vaginal penetration again (it won't be), or that it might look different and put their partner off (it might look different, but fears about the impact of this are usually unfounded). These concerns are not just experienced by people who have

given birth. Partners who were present at births (or just saw or heard about the discomfort their partner was in afterwards) can also feel worried about what their partner's body (or mind) has gone through, and this can impact on their own feelings about sex or their motivation to have it.

Something that can really help here is to talk to your partner about how you feel and any fears you have about what might happen or what they might think, as it's likely that it matters less to them than it does to you. This reassurance can be vital for when you do feel like being sexual again. Talking about such personal fears can be challenging, as many people tell me that they don't want to draw attention to them in case it turns their partner off. The irony is that sharing these fears can do the opposite, allowing you both to relax and enjoy sex without the worry of what the other is thinking or what could go wrong.

Sex is often a way to connect, to feel wanted, to create moments of intimacy and to create a strong emotional climate in a relationship, helping us feel like a team. Sexual satisfaction contributes to relationship satisfaction, so at some point it can be useful to see how becoming parents has knocked you off track and to make some small changes to get things back on a more favourable trajectory – a guide to how to do this is in my book, *How Not to Let Having Kids Ruin Your Sex Life* (2024).

In the first year or so after birth, though, I urge you to give yourselves a break from worrying about your sex life, although do try to keep talking. Try not to let all sexual currency disappear, but remember: sex does not have to include penetrative sex. In fact, there's a whole world of sex available to you without it. If you do manage to find a miraculous window between naps, nappies and feeding when you feel like doing it, remember that desire often won't be present but will need to be kickstarted, and this is normal (it does not mean there's a problem with you or your relationship). Use plenty of lube, and if you're not feeling like it, don't worry too much. At some point you will have the time and inclination to work at it again, and as long as you've kept some element of intimacy, connection and comfort with each other and kept talking, you'll be able to get things back on track. Pay attention to sleep and your psychological wellbeing, as these will lay the foundation for returning to a more satisfying sex life when you feel ready.

Sharing your fears allows you both to relax and enjoy sex without the worry of what the other is thinking or what could go wrong.

LOOK AFTER YOU!

Alongside looking after your baby, which I know will feel like the most important thing in the world at the moment, it is also really, really important that you take care of yourself, so that you can take care of your baby. Hopefully, you will have friends and relatives and partners nearby, or with you, to help support you at this time, but these are the things I really believe you need to pay attention to amid all the nappy changing and feeding:

Nourish yourself

Try to eat as healthily as possible. This is going to help with everything: your mood, your milk supply, your recovery. It will help with sleep, too. Dr Federica has outlined your nutritional needs and the best way to look after your body during the fourth trimester, so please do turn to that section (on page 298) and follow her brilliant advice.

Wash

I know it might sound ridiculous, but you need to bathe and wash your hair, and clean your clothes and change your pad. Self-care is really important for your health and sense of wellbeing, and yet sometimes you can just get so tired or preoccupied with trying to be a good mother that it falls by the wayside. But remember, all of these things are important to prevent infections, and just to help you feel good in and about yourself.

Move gently and get outside

Once you've done your bedrest (see page 257) and are ready to face the world, it's really nice to get outside, breathe some fresh air and go for little walks with your baby. And there are so many mental and physical benefits to this – PT Emma Jeffery talks on page 290; she has so much advice to share if you're keen to get back into movement – and why you should.

Take care of your pelvic floor

Remember those exercises? Turn to page 246 for all Jenny Gillespie's advice.

Laugh, dance, boost your mood

I used to love listening to music. For me, music is like a mood-altering drug. I'd sometimes put on some music and dance with each of my babies and sing – those kinds of things would keep me happy and in a good mood. But do whatever you enjoy, whatever makes you feel good or makes you laugh. And please do try to be aware of your mood, and talk to someone if you're not feeling happy.

When you're a parent, you think you should be absolutely over the moon all the time because you've had a baby, but if you're feeling down or you're struggling, please let the midwife know – they will come and ask you questions, and please try to be honest with yourself and them when you answer. (For more advice on this and where to get help, see pages 276, 311.)

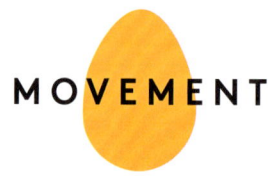

MOVEMENT

I started doing gentle exercise about six weeks after I had Tilly and Chester, and I was extremely careful with the movement that I did. This is important because your tummy muscles are vulnerable, which is why we've asked the wonderful personal trainer Emma Jeffery to talk about how, when and why to get back into movement after birth. And on page 297, we've also asked Tessa Clemson to talk about the benefits of postpartum yoga.

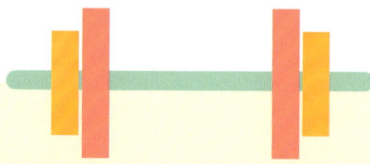

POSTPARTUM MOVEMENT

Emma Jeffery, Personal Trainer

Think of your return to exercise as a three-stage process:

— **Stage one:** In the first six weeks, the focus is on healing and gentle movement to aid your recovery from birth.

— **Stage two:** This stage, following your six-week GP check-up, is about more structured movement, maybe a postnatal programme or class, or working directly with a personal trainer. It's here you will incorporate suitable exercise to strengthen your whole body and help you manage the physical demands of motherhood.

— **Stage three:** This is a continued, graded return to exercise, building on those foundations from the earlier months.

I can't emphasise enough how important it is to invest time and energy in understanding and mastering these components of postpartum 'exercise', as they are the foundation for your postnatal recovery and getting you back to the exercise you love and want to participate in.

I haven't attached any timelines to stages two and three because there really is no one-size-fits-all approach in returning to exercise postpartum. Your journey will be completely unique, and this will influence when and how you feel ready to move. Some of us may need a more tailored approach than is detailed here, but this should give you a reliable overview.

Before diving into the what and the how, here are my top tips for managing your mindset and expectations postpartum:

— Your workouts may not look perfect. You may not be able to work out for the amount of time you hope to, making you feel like you are not getting enough done.

— What works one week may not work the next as your baby's needs and sleep cycles change, or they become more mobile.

— Give yourself permission to adapt, and drop any comparison with others in these early months, because the general consensus is that 12 to 18 months is a realistic timeframe to recover from having a baby.

— Even if you only manage ten minutes of gentle movement each day, it will still be really beneficial. This journey may not be as linear as you imagine or as quick as you want it to be, but there's no need to rush to try to compensate for this. Taking your time will prevent you running into setbacks later.

STAGE ONE

To be clear, in the first six weeks, you will not be doing exercise as you may typically think of it. This stage involves restorative movement, which will help you reconnect with your body. With the right knowledge and expertise, this is actually a period of amazing potential, which can accelerate your healing, especially if you have had an episiotomy, tear or C-section.

First of all, it includes breathwork. It cannot be underestimated how important it is to learn how to breathe well – and this is not just diaphragmatic breathing, but learning how to expand and create space in the whole of the ribcage and using the breath to stretch the intercostal muscles between your ribs. This can help bring about lasting change and is fantastic for regulating your nervous system. It works by creating more space in the top of the ribcage, which in turn takes the pressure off your pelvic floor. This has huge benefits in treating incontinence and prolapse, and the great news is that it can take just five minutes a day and be done in front of the telly.

You can also begin to strengthen your pelvic floor in these early days. This should be considered part of your core recovery, as it sits at the bottom of the abdominal cavity, and just like your core, it needs to be rehabilitated with a graded return to exercise. Lots of women will experience pelvic health issues after having their children, but that doesn't mean they should have to put up with them (see page 243). The great news is that the pelvic floor can be adapted, just like any other muscle in your body. Your starting point is to do your pelvic-floor exercises (or Kegels), and these can start the day after giving birth, or as soon as you feel ready. If you are unsure how to carry these out, see Jenny Gillespie's advice on page 246 or look for guidance on the Squeezy App or website, or reach out to a pelvic health physiotherapist or postnatal personal trainer. It's recommended that these are carried out in a lying-down or side-lying position to begin with, and once you have mastered those you can

move on to performing them sitting and standing.

Stage one can also include going for short walks (or shuffles may be more appropriate) when you feel ready, understanding how your body's alignment and balance has changed, reconnecting to your feet, starting gentle movement (including deep abdominal activation), and building up to movement patterns you are likely to use every day as a parent, like squats and lunges. This will help you feel stronger and more capable, and encourage a deeper understanding of your postnatal body when you join a postnatal-specific exercise class in stage two.

STAGE TWO

If you've had an uncomplicated vaginal delivery, feel well, your scars (if applicable) are healing as expected and postpartum bleeding has stopped, it's likely you will be cleared to return to exercise by your GP at your six-week check-up. If you have had a C-section, the recommendation is to return to exercise slightly later, at least 8 weeks postpartum, maybe later depending on how you are healing. Although many mums see this GP check as a 'green light' to return to exercise, I highly recommend booking a private consultation with a specialist women's

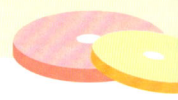

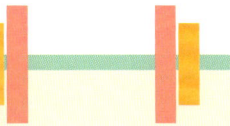

health physiotherapist around this time (postnatal specialists in postpartum physical recovery) to give you a true picture of how your abdominals and pelvic floor are healing. If a private consultation is not an option and you have concerns about how you are recovering beyond the six-week check, do not hesitate to seek support from your GP, who should refer you to a suitable women's health physiotherapist through the NHS.

Assuming all is well, after your GP check, you are looking to make a graded return to exercise, ideally with a suitably qualified postnatal coach. This means working steadily, firstly to build the strength and endurance to meet the demands of being a mum by building core and pelvic-floor foundations and mastering functional movement patterns. This includes squatting, lunging, pushing, pulling, rotating, lifting and carrying; the movements that life asks of us repeatedly as mothers! At the same time, it's important to understand how your body manages pressure and to build up to more dynamic movements, like running and jumping, at a rate that is suited to your body.

In terms of specific core recovery, one of the biggest tips I can give you is to think of it as part of strengthening your whole body, not in isolation. All the

functional movement patterns I mentioned above are core exercises. You may start with strengthening the deep abdominals (transverse abdominis, or TVA) and pelvic floor by lying on your back, but motherhood happens on your feet in the twisting and turning of everyday life, so in time your training should replicate that.

Many people have given up on their pelvic-floor exercises by this stage because they find them boring and don't feel the benefits quickly enough, but just because you can't see the effects immediately, please don't give up. They are working, and most people feel the benefits of committing to a pelvic-floor strengthening programme within 12 weeks.

STAGE THREE

During stage three, you will continue to build on the strengthening movements you have been working on in the earlier stages. This will include gradually increasing the weights you are using and following a programme that helps you return to higher impact exercise appropriately.

The best strategy to strengthen any muscle, including your abdominals, is to challenge them. Using progressively heavier weights or more challenging movements (known as progressive overload) is the key to bringing about muscular change. Doing abdominal exercises that are too easy, and sticking with them for too long, does not tend to create the changes most of my clients are seeking. These changes take time and consistency, but you can achieve them much more quickly if you work with a progressive postnatal coach who understands your body, how to challenge you appropriately and adapt your movement patterns to keep you moving forward in empowering ways.

What is needed in addition to your pelvic-floor exercises at this stage is a strategy that includes movement. That plan should include progressive overload and full-body approach, which looks to strengthen your glutes, hips, legs and core – all of which play a wider role in supporting the pelvic floor. It's important to learn techniques that teach you how to create more length, space and range of movement in and around the pelvis, which houses your pelvic floor and also helps you manage abdominal pressure better by looking at your posture and breathing.

Many women avoid certain movements through fear of making any pelvic health symptoms worse, but I would say from experience, it's typically these movements that are the very thing you need and the missing piece in the puzzle of your recovery. This is particularly the case with jumping and running. Your training programme should also help you learn how to build up to more explosive movements, let go of unnecessary tension and also absorb impact from these types of activities. So, working out standing up on your feet is really important; you should not feel restricted to mat-based exercises.

I do not want to curb your enthusiasm for more high impact activities like running. Running is popular with my postnatal clients as it's accessible, is a fantastic stress-reliever and gets those endorphins circulating. But running is an impactful exercise. What this means is that you will need a focused, progressive training programme that will help strengthen your whole body, from the foot up, and is respectful of your pelvic-floor (see the resources on page 310). It is advised that you do not return to running, without guidance from a pelvic health physiotherapist and support from an appropriately qualified postnatal personal trainer if you are experiencing any symptoms of pelvic health dysfunction.

When you have strategies that help you understand why you are experiencing pelvic-floor-related symptoms from a whole-body perspective, you will have a greater chance of recovering faster and keeping those symptoms at bay.

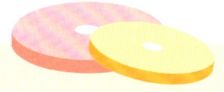

ABDOMINAL SEPARATION

Emma Jeffery, Personal Trainer

Many of the mums I work with ask me about abdominal separation (also known as diastasis recti abdominis, or DRA), so I want to reassure you that every mum will experience this by the third trimester. It is a normal, natural adaptation and everyone will recover differently. Abdominal separation specifically refers to the widening and thinning of the linea alba – this is the long, vertical line of connective tissue that separates your rectus muscles (your six-pack muscles), which sometimes darkens during pregnancy. It does not refer to a muscle that has separated, which is a common misconception.

The combination of an abdominal gap and a loss of tension through the linea alba may mean that some of you will see doming or a ridge through your midline when doing something your body finds challenging, like moving from lying down to sitting up, or lifting something overhead or heavy. This is to do with how your core is managing pressure within your abdominal cavity, and it dictates how a movement or exercise may need modifying.

The only time you need specifically to adapt or find a new movement strategy is if the ridge or doming is hard when you perform an exercise. If that hard ridge stays when you try to push it back down, it's a sign that this specific movement has exceeded the threshold that your body is able to handle at this stage. This not only applies to exercising. You may also notice your abdomen doming when carrying out day-to-day activities, such as lifting the pushchair, the car seat or older children – as mothers we are lifting all the time! If the doming is soft, you are generally okay to perform that movement; if it is hard then, for now, you need a different strategy to help your body manage that pressure.

This is when you need to seek advice from a postnatal personal trainer or women's health physiotherapist. A strategy may be as simple as bringing your attention to your lifting technique, helping you understand how to get a good inhale and use a good exhale, and to check you are actually using your feet effectively to generate force upwards and not bearing down. Of course, if you have any concerns whatsoever, please seek advice from your GP and ask for a referral to a specialist women's health physiotherapist.

The approach I've described here is likely to be more involved than many mums expect; it goes beyond just pelvic-floor exercises and a few specific core exercises, and may take longer than anticipated. This is because, for a long time, mums haven't received the right information they need on how to care for their postpartum bodies. Thankfully this is now changing, slowly, and there are now lots of postnatal exercise programmes available, which will provide you with all the guidance I have spoken about here, and offer you a whole host of other movement-related benefits such as strength building and cardiovascular endurance, plus those important mood-boosting, endorphin-related highs.

Your recovery is completely individual to you, your birth and your postpartum experiences. It's okay for the timeframes I've mentioned here to shift, depending on how ready you feel, and of course this could change day by day. It also depends on the amount of rest/sleep you are able to get, your nutrition, your mental wellbeing, the support you have around you and the steps you are able to take to rehabilitate your body.

Remember to listen to your body, meet yourself with compassion and celebrate every single moment you are able to dedicate to your postnatal recovery – it really does all add up!

> **Remember to listen to your body, meet yourself with compassion and celebrate every single moment you are able to dedicate to your postnatal recovery.**

POSTPARTUM YOGA

Tessa Clemson, Yoga Teacher

Yoga prepares us physically and mentally for the postpartum period – a time of healing, recovery and restoration. Gentle stretches optimise the pelvic floor and help your body to heal slowly, building core strength and preventing symptoms such as diastasis recti (separation of the abdominal muscles).

Deeper stretches help to relieve achy muscles from lifting, feeding and holding babies, or sleeping in awkward positions. Continuing to prioritise your health and wellbeing sets a great example to your baby, too.

Wait until you are six weeks postnatal and have had your GP check if you have had a vaginal birth, or ten weeks if you've had a caesarean birth, before starting to practise. The beauty of yoga is that it can be done anywhere, at any time, and you don't need lots of equipment. Whether you are practising online or you have a yoga class local to you, make sure the teacher is fully trained and insured, and let them know that you are postnatal, as the exercises may

need to be adapted. Any trauma to the perineum must be fully healed before attending a yoga class unless it is specifically postnatal. Always seek advice from a health practitioner if you have any questions or concerns.

Try to find a class, teacher and style that resonates with you. A night class might improve your sleep, or a gentle morning stretch might set you up for the day – it is your practice and your journey, so be open to finding what suits you, your body and your baby.

Look out for classes that have a community that feels supportive, welcoming and informed. Sessions should not be too strenuous, and you should stay cool and hydrated.

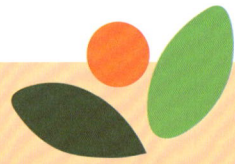

POSTPARTUM NUTRITION

Dr Federica Amati, Nutritionist

The three months after birth are often described as the fourth trimester. Mother and baby are so biologically linked at this time that it's also common to refer to them as 'the mother–baby dyad', i.e. not really separate entities, and any mother can likely confirm that when their newborn baby cries, there is a deep, cellular response urging them to do something. In my experience, that biological response can sometimes lead to mums forgetting to nourish themselves at a time when their bodies and minds, as well as their sense of self, are undergoing a seismic shift. Giving birth is a physical trauma, which, though natural, still requires a recovery period, and for that the body needs sustenance.

The body undergoes an enormous metabolic and physiological shift during pregnancy, building new organs and tissues as well as a whole new human, which is then birthed with a combination of blood, sweat and tears, and a huge rollercoaster of hormonal changes to follow. Our nutritional needs then shift postpartum from building and strengthening to repairing and

protecting. Repairing tissue damage calls for foods that are high in good-quality proteins, as well as fruits and vegetables that contain antioxidants and vitamins, such as vitamin C. Iron-rich foods, including beans, lentils, eggs, fish and meat, can help replenish any lost blood, which may have worsened our iron status.

One of the most obvious consequences of having a newborn is broken, irregular sleep and often feeling exhausted; this might call for caffeinated coffee to make its return to our lives, which is, luckily, safe in normal amounts (one to three cups per day) if you are breastfeeding. One note of caution here, however, is that if your baby is very sensitive to coffee (we all have different tolerance levels), it may disturb their sleep. Drinking coffee in the morning might save you from having a very alert baby at bedtime.

Drinking alcohol during breastfeeding has a much less direct impact on the baby's development than it does in pregnancy, but its effect on a sleep-deprived parent can be a problem.

With a newborn to look after, having more than one drink can result in the night feeds and the next day being even harder on you, and potentially dangerous for the baby if you are less alert when you're feeding them, regardless of how you are feeding them.

Most of the fat stored in pregnancy is designated to be used for breastmilk directly, which is handy as it is energetically demanding work. Breastfeeding mothers require more energy (roughly 500 extra calories per day) than those who don't breastfeed, and they also need to pay more attention to staying hydrated. What a mother eats also impacts her breastmilk's composition in terms of micronutrient content and flavour: eating garlic, spices and fresh herbs will increase the number of nutrients your baby receives, as well as vary the flavour of the breastmilk, helping them develop a more diverse palate. The only supplement recommended for breastfeeding mothers is vitamin D, which only needs to be supplemented in the winter months, or if you spend less than 20 minutes per day with sunlight on your skin, at the recommended dose of 10 mcg (400 IUD) per day.

For mothers who can't or choose not to breastfeed, understanding the rapid change in hormones and often very quick return to regular menstrual cycles is key. Recovery from birth remains the priority, but there is no need for additional energy as there is when breastfeeding, and some of the pregnancy weight gained as stores for breastfeeding could persist for longer than it does with breastfeeding mothers.

Regardless of how you feed your baby, supporting yourself through this unique period of readjustment in your life is crucial. Eating plenty of fibre-rich foods, nourishing meals and foods that reduce inflammation, such as colourful berries, leafy greens and legumes, yoghurt, kefir and other fermented foods, can hugely improve your energy levels and sleep quality, and reduce the inflammation resulting from birth and the temporary loss of sleep.

Our cultural environment makes it too easy to reach for packaged snacks, energy drinks and foods like cookies, sweets and soft drinks, but these won't benefit you or your baby in the short or long term. I often recommend making lots of healthy meals and ready-to-go snacks – such as veg-packed burritos, fish pie, vegetable lasagne, dates with almonds and dark chocolate, trail mix, frozen-berry yoghurt pots or home-baked high-fibre cookies – in the weeks before birth so that you have easy options when you won't have as much time to cook from scratch.

Below you'll find some meal ideas tailored to each stage of pregnancy, featuring Mediterranean-inspired choices to help you create delicious, balanced dishes that will nourish you and your growing baby.

Breakfast

FIRST TRIMESTER

Natural yoghurt with fresh berries and nuts;

or

wholegrain bread with avocado, butter beans, tomato and extra virgin olive oil

SECOND TRIMESTER

Organic oatmeal with chopped nuts, flaxseed and fresh or frozen fruit;

or

smoothie with spinach, banana, kefir, nut butter and chia seeds;

or

wholegrain bagel with avocado or smashed peas, fresh herbs, lemon and smoked salmon

THIRD TRIMESTER

Scrambled eggs with spinach, mushrooms and feta cheese served with farinata (chickpea flatbread) or a wholemeal sourdough

Mid-morning snack

FIRST TRIMESTER

Almonds and a piece of fruit (e.g. an apple or pear);

or

a frozen blueberry, banana, kefir, almond butter and spinach smoothie

SECOND TRIMESTER

Handful of walnuts and dried apricots

THIRD TRIMESTER

Natural yoghurt with a handful of mixed berries and a spoonful of nut butter

Lunch

FIRST TRIMESTER

Quinoa or spelt salad with chickpeas, cucumber, tomatoes and feta cheese, plus mixed leafy greens with olive oil and lemon dressing

SECOND TRIMESTER

Wholegrain pita bread with falafel, hummus and mixed greens, tomato and cucumber salad with olive oil and fresh herbs

THIRD TRIMESTER

Lentils and chopped greens with durum wheat or legume pasta, chopped salad with avocado, olives, cherry tomatoes, and extra virgin olive oil dressing

Afternoon snack

FIRST TRIMESTER

Carrot and celery sticks with hummus

SECOND TRIMESTER

Edamame beans

THIRD TRIMESTER

Apple slices with almond butter

Dinner

FIRST TRIMESTER

Lentil and vegetable stew with wholegrain bread; steamed broccoli and spinach served with salmon or mackerel

SECOND TRIMESTER

Stuffed peppers with barley, black beans, corn and tomatoes, roasted Brussels sprouts and sweet potatoes

THIRD TRIMESTER

Salmon or tofu bake with broccoli, greens, peas, carrots and beetroot served with pearl barley

Evening snack

FIRST TRIMESTER

SECOND TRIMESTER

Fruit salad with a sprinkle of pumpkin seeds and a square of dark chocolate

THIRD TRIMESTER

Chia pudding with your favourite milk, almonds and fresh mango

ONE LAST THING BEFORE THE BIRTHING ADVENTURES BEGIN

I don't think that there is a moment in a woman's life when she is more powerful and yet more vulnerable than when she gets pregnant, right up until the time she's given birth, and even for the six months afterwards. This is the time when women need to be empowered and cared for in equal measure. They need to be heard, supported, loved, encouraged and informed.

Because when women are afforded all of these things, they feel safe, and that is going to have a really positive impact on their birthing experience. I feel so strongly that we OWE it to pregnant women and labouring mothers to make this time in their lives as beautiful and as empowering as possible.

But what I've witnessed in the 24 years since I first became pregnant, is a gradual erosion of pregnant and birthing women's rights and their access to the care they deserve. Many women are being disempowered: their control and autonomy is being removed; they are being misinformed so that their labour can be sped up or for a ward to be cleared; or they're not having their birth preferences honoured because there's no space at the birthing centre or stretched medical staff don't have the capacity to respect their wishes. This has to change.

Giving birth is a very, very important time in a woman's life and we all need to work to ensure that they are given the best chances of having a positive birth experience. Because even in an emergency, that IS possible. It doesn't come down to the style of birth. As we've shown, there's no way of knowing which type of birth will suit you and your baby until you're in the moment. But the way women are spoken to, the way they are made to understand their choices, and whether they are made to feel in control of their situation can change their entire experience of birth. And this is why I love amazing midwives. Midwives are the people who can enable an empowered birth, so I just want to say thank you to all the midwives who work so tirelessly to make giving birth a special experience.

The thing I hear time and time again is that being heard, being seen, being understood, being respected, makes the world of difference. And I wanted to provide a book that would give you all the information and tools for you to seek and receive the birth that you deserve – and if you can't have that birth, then the best version of the birth you weren't expecting.

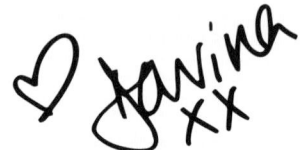

Please remember: you are a magical vessel. You are bringing life into the world.

You are beautiful, you are brave and you are strong.

Love you x

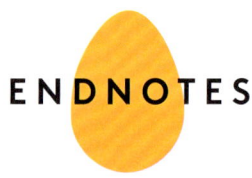

ENDNOTES

1   'Diagnosis: Infertility', NHS: https://www.nhs.uk/conditions/infertility/diagnosis/

2   Kurt T. Barnhart and Courtney A. Schreiber, 'Return to fertility following discontinuation of oral contraceptives', *Fertility and Sterility*, 91(3), 2009, 659–63: DOI: 10.1016/j.fertnstert.2009.01.003

3   Fadi Yahya, 'Infertility and Stress', Mayo Clinic Health System, 24 August 2022: https://www.mayoclinichealthsystem.org/hometown-health/speaking-of-health/infertility-and-stress#

4   Elizabeth Scott, 'Want to Relieve Stress ASAP? Write in a Gratitude Journal', Verywell Mind, 11 September 2023: https://www.verywellmind.com/writing-in-a-gratitude-journal-for-stress-relief-3144887

5   https://www.healthline.com/health/mental-health/can-shaking-your-body-heal-stress-and-trauma

6   Rosalba Courtney et al., 'Relationship between dysfunctional breathing patterns and ability to achieve target heart rate variability with features of "coherence" during biofeedback', *Alternative Therapies in Health and Medicine*, May–June 2011, 17(3), 38–44. PMID: 22164811.

7   Grace Pien and Richard Schwab, 'Sleep disorders during pregnancy', *Sleep,* 1 November 2004, 27(7), 1405–17. DOI: 10.1093/sleep/27.7.1405. PMID: 15586794

8   Liwen Li et al., 'Association between Sleep-Disordered Breathing during Pregnancy and Maternal and Fetal Outcomes: An Updated Systematic Review and Meta-Analysis', *Frontiers in Neurology*, 28 May 2018, 9(91). DOI: 10.3389/fneur.2018.00091. PMID: 29892255; PMCID: PMC5985400.

9   Nicole Brown et al., 'The intrapartum and perinatal risks of sleep-disordered breathing in pregnancy: a systematic review and metaanalysis', *American Journal of Obstetrics and Gynecology*, August 2018, 219(2), 147–161. DOI: 10.1016/j.ajog.2018.02.004. Epub 15 February 2018. PMID: 29454869.

10 Francesca Facco et al., 'Association Between Sleep-Disordered Breathing and Hypertensive Disorders of Pregnancy and Gestational Diabetes Mellitus', *Obstetrics & Gynecology*, January 2017, 129(1), 31–41. DOI: 10.1097/AOG.0000000000001805. PMID: 27926645; PMCID: PMC5512455.

11 Jennifer Dominguez et al., 'Society of Anesthesia and Sleep Medicine and the Society for Obstetric Anesthesia and Perinatology Consensus Guideline on the Screening, Diagnosis, and Treatment of Obstructive Sleep Apnea in Pregnancy', *Obstetrics & Gynecology*, 1 August 2023, 142(2), 403–23. DOI: 10.1097/AOG.0000000000005261. Epub 5 July 2023. PMID: 37411038; PMCID: PMC10351908.

12 Alex Perkins and Alys Einion, 'Pregnant pause: should we screen for sleep disordered breathing in pregnancy?' *Breathe* (Sheff), March 2019, 15(1), 36–44. DOI: 10.1183/20734735.0343-2018. PMID: 30838058; PMCID: PMC6395990.

13 Sabina Tim and Agnieszka Mazur-Bialy, 'The Most Common Functional Disorders and Factors Affecting Female Pelvic Floor', *Life* (Basel),

14 December 2021, 11(12), 1397. DOI: 10.3390/life11121397. PMID: 34947928; PMCID: PMC8704638.

14 Fadi Yahya, 'Infertility and Stress', Mayo Clinic Health System, 24 August 2022: https://www.mayoclinichealthsystem.org/hometown-health/speaking-of-health/infertility-and-stress#

15 'Vitamins, supplements and nutrition in pregnancy', NHS: https://www.nhs.uk/pregnancy/keeping-well/vitamins-supplements-and-nutrition/ (accessed 25 June 2024).

16 'Next baby: What does high risk mean?', NHS: https://www.bsuh.nhs.uk/maternity/wp-content/uploads/sites/7/2016/09/Next-baby-info.pdf (accessed 24 June 2024).

17 'Causes of gestational diabetes', Diabetes UK: https://www.diabetes.org.uk/diabetes-the-basics/gestational-diabetes/causes#

18 https://www.npeu.ox.ac.uk/assets/downloads/mbrrace-uk/reports/maternal-report-2024/MBRRACE-UK_Maternal_Report_2024%20_Lay_Summary_V1.0.pdf

19 https://www.npeu.ox.ac.uk/assets/downloads/mbrrace-uk/reports/MBRRACE-UK%20Maternal%20Report%202018%20-%20Lay%20Summary%20v1.0.pdf

20 https://pubmed.ncbi.nlm.nih.gov/15180027/#:~:text=Abstract,surgeon%2C%20teacher%2C%20and%20writer.

21 https://www.bbc.co.uk/news/blogs-trending-41692593

https://www.nursingtimes.net/news/education/racist-nursing-textbook-pulled-after-criticism-on-social-media-26-10-2017/

22 https://www.ncbi.nlm.nih.gov/pmc/articles/PMC4843483/

23 https://www.bmj.com/content/378/bmj.o2337

24 https://www.npeu.ox.ac.uk/mbrrace-uk/reports

25 https://webarchive.nationalarchives.gov.uk/ukgwa/20030801172235/http://www.doh.gov.uk:80/cmo/mdeaths.htm#summary%20of%20key%20findings

26 https://fivexmore.org/blackmereport

27 https://hansard.parliament.uk/Commons/2021-04-19/debates/6935B9C7-6419-4E7B-A813-E852A4EE4F5C/BlackMaternalHealthcareAndMortality

28 https://fivexmore.org/blackmereport

29 'Miscarriage statistics', Tommy's: https://www.tommys.org/baby-loss-support/miscarriage-information-and-support/miscarriage-statistics

30 'Causes: Miscarriage', NHS: https://www.nhs.uk/conditions/miscarriage/causes/

31 'Where to give birth: the options', NHS: https://www.nhs.uk/pregnancy/labour-and-birth/preparing-for-the-birth/where-to-give-birth-the-options/ (accessed 20 April 2024).

32 Andry Vleeming et al., A., 'European guidelines for the diagnosis and treatment of pelvic girdle pain', *European Spine Journal,* 17(6), 8 February 2008, 794–819, DOI: 10.1007/s00586-008-0602-4

33 'Pelvic pain in pregnancy', NHS: https://www.nhs.uk/pregnancy/related-conditions/common-symptoms/pelvic-pain/

34 A. Frankam et al., 'Pregnancy related pelvic girdle pain: the influence of pain science on the understanding of its causes and treatment choices', *Pelvic Obstetric & Gynaecological Physiotherapy,* 132, spring 2023, 49–60.

35   Esther van Benten et al., 'Recommendations for physical therapists on the treatment of lumbopelvic pain during pregnancy; a systematic review', *Journal of Orthopaedic Sports and Physical Therapy,* 44(7), 10 May 2014, 464–73, DOI: 10.2519/jospt.2014.5098

36   Susan Clinton et al., 'Pelvic girdle pain in the antepartum population: Physical therapy clinical practice guidelines linked to the international classification of functioning, disability, and health from the section on women's health and the orthopaedic section of the American Physical Therapy Association', *Journal of Women's Health Physical Therapy*, 41(2), May 2017, 102–25, DOI: 10.1097/JWH.0000000000000081

37   A. Simonds et al., 'Clinical practice guidelines for pelvic girdle pain in the postpartum population', *Journal of Women's Health Physical Therapy,* 46, 1 January 2022, E1–E38, DOI:10.1097/jwh.0000000000000236

38   Sheena Byrom and Soo Downe, *Squaring the Circle: Normal Birth Research, Theory and Practice in a Technological Age* (London: Pinter & Martin Limited, 2019), 60.

39   'Exercising in pregnancy', NHS Start for Life: www.nhs.uk/start-for-life/pregnancy/exercising-in-pregnancy (accessed 26 June 2024).

40   Kylie Rymanowicz, 'Infant vision development: Helping babies see their bright futures!' Michigan State University Extension, 18 December 2014: https://www.canr.msu.edu/news/infant_vision_development_helping_babies_see_their_bright_futures

41   e-Library of Evidence for Nutrition Actions (eLENA), 'Optimal timing of cord clamping for the prevention of iron deficiency anaemia in infants', World Health Organization, 9 August 2023: https://www.who.int/tools/elena/interventions/cord-clamping

42   Ola Andersson and Judith Mercer, 'Cord Management of the Term Newborn', *Clinics in Perinatology*, 48(3), August 2021, 447–470. DOI: 10.1016/j.clp.2021.05.002

43   Leanne Jones et al., 'Pain management for women in labour: an overview of systematic reviews', Cochrane Database of Systematic Reviews 2012, (3), Article CD009234, 12 March 2012. DOI: 10.1002/14651858.CD009234.pub2; Leyla Mollamahmutoğlu et al., 'The effects of immersion in water on labor, birth and newborn and comparison with epidural analgesia and conventional vaginal delivery', *Journal of the Turkish-German Gynecological Association,* 13(1), 1 March 2012, 45–9. DOI: 10.5152/jtgga.2012.03. PMID: 24627674; PMCID: PMC3940223

44   The Bishop score is a scoring system used to decide how likely it is that you will go into labour soon. A midwife will carry out a vaginal examination to assess the cervix – its softness, position, length and how open it is – and how deep your baby's head is in the pelvis. Each factor is given a value, which are then added up to give you an overall score that is used to determine whether they should recommend induction, and how likely it is that an induction will result in a vaginal birth.

45   'Skin-to-skin contact', UNICEF: https://www.unicef.org.uk/babyfriendly/baby-friendly-resources/implementing-standards-resources/skin-to-skin-contact/ (accessed 29 July 2024).

46   Information taken from 'Skin-to-skin contact', UNICEF: https://www.unicef. org.uk/babyfriendly/baby-friendly-resources/implementing-standards-resources/skin-to-skin-contact/ (accessed 29 July 2024).

47   Hans Dietz, 'Pelvic floor trauma in childbirth', *Australian & New Zealand Journal of Obstetrics & Gynaecology,* 53(3), June 2013, 220–230. DOI: 10.1111/ajo.12059.

48   Carlina Deflorin et al., 'Physical management of scar tissue; A systematic review and meta-analysis', *Journal of Alternative and Complementary Medicine*, 26(10), October 2020, 854–865. DOI: 10.1089/acm.2020.0109.

49   Lisa Kim et al., 'Pelvic Health Physical Therapy Improves Pelvic Floor Women with Obstetric Anal Sphincter Injuries', *Journal of Women's Health Physical Therapy*, 46(1), January 2022, 18–24. DOI: 10.1097/JWH.0000000000000223

50   Kari Bø, 'Physiotherapy management of urinary incontinence in females', *Australian Journal of Physiotherapy*, 66(3), July 2020, 147–154. DOI: 10.1016/j.jphys.2020.06.011

51   Suzanne Hagen et al., 'Individualised pelvic floor muscle training in women with pelvic organ prolapse; A multicentre randomised control trial', *The Lancet*, 383(9919), 1 March 2014; 796–806. DOI: 10.1016/S0140-6736(13)61977-7

52   E. Hoekzema et al.(2017). Pregnancy Leads to Long-lasting Changes in Human Brain Structure, *Nature Neuroscience* 20, pp287–296.

53   'Body image in adulthood', Mental Health Foundation: https://www.mentalhealth.org.uk/our-work/research/body-image-how-we-think-and-feel-about-our-bodies/body-image-adulthood

54   Natalie O. Rosen et al., 'Unmet and Exceeded Expectations for Sexual Concerns across the Transition to Parenthood', *Journal of Sex Research*, 60(9), 2023, 1235–46. DOI: 10.1080/00224499.2022.2126814; Tone Ahlborg et al., 'Quality of the intimate and sexual relationship in first-time parents six months after delivery', *Journal of Sex Research,* 42(2), 2005, 167–74. DOI: 10.1080/00224490509552270

55   Hera Schlagintweit et al., 'A new baby in the bedroom: Frequency and severity of postpartum sexual concerns and their associations with relationship satisfaction in new parent couples', *Journal of Sexual Medicine,* 13(10), 2016, 1455–65. DOI: 10.1016/j.jsxm.2016.08.006

56   G. Barrett et al., 'Women's sexual health after childbirth', *British Journal of Obstetrics and Gynaecology,* 107, 2000, 186–19. DOI: 10.1111/j.1471-0528.2000.tb11689.x

57   Sofia Jawed-Wessel and Emily Sevick, 'The Impact of Pregnancy and Childbirth on Sexual Behaviors: A Systematic Review', *Journal of Sex Research,* 54(4–5), 2017, 411–23. DOI: 10.1080/00224499.2016.1274715

58   Ibid

59   Lauren Hipp et al., 'Exploring women's postpartum sexuality: social, psychological, relational, and birth-related contextual factors', *Journal of Sexual Medicine,* 9(9), 2012, 2330–41. DOI: 10.1111/j.1743-6109.2012.02804.x

60   David Kalmbach et al., 'The impact of sleep on female sexual response and behavior: A pilot study', *Journal of Sexual Medicine*, 12(5), 2015, 1221–32. DOI: 10.1111/jsm.12858

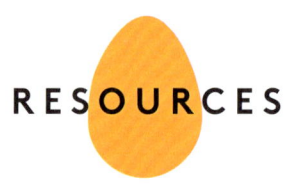

RESOURCES

GENERAL HEALTH ADVICE AND FORUMS

Health Canada
canada.ca/en/health-canada.html

Healthdirect Australia
healthdirect.gov.au

HealthUnlocked healthunlocked.com

HSE about.hse.ie

Mayo Clinic mayoclinic.org

MedlinePlus medlineplus.gov/
pregnancy.html

National Institute for Health and Care
Excellence nice.org.uk

NHS nhs.u

NHS inform nhsinform.scot

NI Direct nidirect.gov.uk

NHS Wales nhs.wales

WebMD webmd.com

GENERAL PERINATAL ADVICE

BabyCentre babycentre.co.uk

Birthrights birthrights.org.uk

Caroline Flint, *Do Birth: A Gentle Guide
to Labour and Childbirth*, The Do Book
Co, 2023

National Childbirth Trust nct.org.uk

Pregnancy Birth and Baby
pregnancybirthbaby.org.au

Raisingchildren.net.au raisingchildren.
net.au

Tommy's tommys.org

ANTENATAL CLASSES

Bump & Baby Club
bumpandbabyclub.com

Happy Parents Happy Baby
happyparentshappybaby.com

NCT nct.org.uk

NowBaby On Demand
nowbaby.co.uk/on-demand

BABIES WITH COMPLEX PARENTING AND MEDICAL NEEDS

Little Miracles
littlemiraclescharity.org.uk

Scope scope.org.uk

**For resources related to raising
children with learning disabilities:**

Mencap mencap.org.uk

BEREAVEMENT

**In the event of a baby loss, you can
access specialist support from
charities such as:**

Baby's Breath babysbreathcanada.ca

Children's Bereavement Center
childbereavement.org/about-us

First Candle firstcandle.org

The Lullaby Trust lullabytrust.org.uk

Petals petalscharity.org

Pregnancy & Infant Loss Support
Centre pilsc.org

Sands sands.org.uk

Saying Goodbye sayinggoodbye.org

Teddy's Wish teddyswish.org

Tommy's (see page 'Baby loss information and support') tommys.org/baby-loss-support

The Worst Girl Gang Ever Foundation theworstgirlgangever.co.uk

Resources related to miscarriage:

The Miscarriage Association miscarriageassociation.org.uk

Miscarriage Australia miscarriageaustralia.com.au

The Pink Elephants Support Network pinkelephants.org.au

Resources related to stillbirth:

International Stillbirth Alliance stillbirthalliance.org

Stillbirth Centre of Research Excellence stillbirthcre.org.au/parents

BIRTH PARTNERS (DOULAS AND MIDWIVES)

Birthrights birthrights.org.uk/factsheets/birth-partners/#choose

Caroline Flint, Sensitive Midwifery: New Edition, Midwifery Gems, 2024

Doula UK doula.org.uk

DONA International dona.org

Ina May Gaskin, *Spiritual Midwifery* – 4th Edition, Book Publishing Company, 2002

Mums and Midwives Awareness Academy mamaacademy.org.uk

BLACK MATERNITY

Five X More fivexmore.org

The Motherhood Group themotherhoodgroup.org/support

Tommy's (see page 'Tommy's Helpline in partnership with Five X More for Black and Black Mixed-Heritage women') tommys.org/pregnancy-information/about-tommys-pregnancy-information/video-call-service

Resources related to Black maternity doulas:

National Black Doulas Association blackdoulas.org

BREATHING

Dr Louise Oliver Therapeutic Life Coaching drlouiseolivertherapeuticlifecoaching.com

CAESAREAN BIRTH AND VBAC

Caesarean caesarean.org.uk

International Caesarean Awareness Network ican-online.org

COMPLICATIONS DURING PREGNANCY

Antenatal Results and Choices arc-uk.org

Fetal Health Foundation fetalhealthfoundation.org

Miracle Babies Foundation miraclebabies.org.au

MoMMAs Voices mommasvoices.org

MotherToBaby mothertobaby.org

ISSUES WITH CONCEIVING AND ASSISTED FERTILITY

American Society for Reproductive Medicine – ReproductiveFacts.org reproductivefacts.org (US)

Fertility Friends Support Forum fertilityfriends.co.uk

Fertility Network UK fertilitynetworkuk.org

Human Fertilisation & Embryology Authority hfea.gov.uk

IVF Babble ivfbabble.com

Resolve: The National Infertility Association resolve.org

Society for Assisted Reproductive Technology sart.org/about-us/what-is-sart

Further reading on egg freezing:

Human Fertilisation & Embryology Authority (see page 'Egg freezing') hfea.gov.uk/treatments/fertility-preservation/egg-freezing

Some fertility tracker apps:

FLO flo.health

Kindara kindara.com

Clue helloclue.com

Relationship support while trying to conceive:

Care for the Family careforthefamily.org.uk

Relate relate.org.uk/about-relate

DRUGS AND ADDICTION

Adfam adfam.org.uk/other-support-services

Frank talktofrank.com/contact-frank

MotherToBaby mothertobaby.org

SMART Recovery smartrecovery.org.uk

EXERCISE DURING AND AFTER PREGNANCY

Absolute.Physio – Gráinne Donnelly (see page 'Advice & Exercise before & after Pregnancy') absolute.physio/advice-exercise-before-after-pregnancy

Active Pregnancy Foundation activepregnancyfoundation.org

GOV.UK (see page 'Guidance: Physical activity guidelines: UK Chief Medical Officers' report') gov.uk/government/publications/physical-activity-guidelines-uk-chief-medical-officers-report

Tessa Clemson Yoga tessaclemsonyoga.com

FEEDING

Association of Breastfeeding Mothers abm.me.uk

The Breastfeeding Network breastfeedingnetwork.org.uk

Breastfeeding Support breastfeeding.support

La Leche League GB laleche.org.uk

National Breastfeeding Helpline nationalbreastfeedinghelpline.org.uk

FERTILITY RESOURCES FOR MEN

Men's Health Forum menshealthforum.org.uk

HIM Fertility himfertility.com

Resources related to fatherhood and miscarriages:

Dad Still Standing dadstillstanding.com

FOOD AND NUTRITION

ZOE (see page 'Pregnancy') zoe.com/learn/category/life-stages/pregnancy

FINANCIAL ADVICE AND SUPPORT

Citizens Advice citizensadvice.org.uk

GOV.UK (see page 'Pregnancy and birth') gov.uk/browse/childcare-parenting/pregnancy-birth

MoneyHelper moneyhelper.org.uk/en

Turn2us benefits-calculator.turn2us.org.uk

Vestpod.com vestpod.com

The Wallet podcast open.spotify.comshow/5nUAIDpJaKf FmzaF5DzYa2

Resources for saving with children:

GOV.UK (see page 'Child Benefit') gov.uk/child-benefit

MoneyHelper (see page 'Saving for your children') moneyhelper.org.uk/en/savings/types-of-savings/saving-for-your-children

FREE/UNASSISTED BIRTH

Birthrights (see page 'Unassisted birth') birthrights.org.uk/factsheets/unassisted-birth

Caroline Flint, *Do Birth: A Gentle Guide to Labour and Childbirth*, The Do Book Co, 2023

HAVING MULTIPLES (E.G. TWINS, TRIPLETS)

Twins Trust twinstrust.org

MATRESCENCE

Matrescence matrescence.uk

Motherkind motherkind.co

MENTAL HEALTH SUPPORT

If you're struggling emotionally, your GP can refer you to a local NHS psychology service if appropriate and advise you on local self-help groups and mental health charities offering support. For crises that present an immediate threat to yourself and/or your baby, call 999 or go to A&E now. You can also receive urgent mental health support through NHS 111 online or by dialling 111.

Centre of Perinatal Excellence cope.org.au/

Gidget Foundation Australia gidgetfoundation.org.au/

Maternal Mental Health Alliance maternalmentalhealthalliance.org/

Mind mind.org.uk/

MumsAid mums-aid.org/

PANDAS pandasfoundation.org.uk/ or call 0808 1961 776

Peach Tree peachtree.org.au/

Royal College of Psychiatrists rcpsych.ac.uk/mental-health

Samaritans samaritans.org/ or call 116 123

Resources for stress during pregnancy:

Anxiety UK anxietyuk.org.uk

Dr Caroline Boyd drcarolineboyd.com

Mental Health Foundation mentalhealth.org.uk

NHS Better Health – Every Mind Matters nhs.uk/every-mind-matters

No Panic nopanic.org.uk

The Stress Management Society stress.org.uk

Resources for birth trauma:

Birth Trauma Association birthtraumaassociation.org

Birth Trauma Australia birthtrauma.org.au

Emma Mills emmamillsmidwife.com

Resources for perinatal obsessive-compulsive disorder:

Maternal OCD maternalocd.org

Resources for postnatal/ postpartum depression:

Association for Post Natal Illness apni.org/ or call 0207 386 0868

ForWhen forwhenhelpline.org.au

PostpartumDepression.org postpartumdepression.org

Postpartum International postpartum.net

Resources for postnatal/ postpartum psychosis:

Action on Postpartum Psychosis app-network.org/ or call 020 33229900

Resources for private talking therapy:

The British Association for Counselling and Psychotherapy bacp.co.uk

The British Psychological Society bps.org.uk

EDMR Association UK emdrassociation.org.uk

Parent Therapy Hub drcarolineboyd.com

The UK Council for Psychotherapy psychotherapy.org.uk

MORNING SICKNESS (HYPEREMESIS GRAVIDARUM)

Pregnancy Sickness Support pregnancysicknesssupport.org.uk

NEONATAL CARE SUPPORT

Miracle Moon miraclemoon.co.uk

PELVIC GIRDLE PAIN

NHS (see page 'Pelvic pain in pregnancy') nhs.uk/pregnancy/related-conditions/common-symptoms/pelvic-pain

The Pelvic Partnership pelvicpartnership.org.uk

Pelvic Obstetric & Gynaecological Physiotherapy (see the POGP booklets) thepogp.co.uk/patient_information/womens_health/pregnancy_pgp_lbp.aspx

Royal College of Obstetricians and Gynaecologists (see page 'Pelvic girdle pain and pregnancy') rcog.org.uk/for-the-public/browse-our-patient-information/pelvic-girdle-pain-and-pregnancy

POSTNATAL RECOVERY

The Mummy Hub themummyhub.com

Pelvic Obstetrics and Gynaecological Physiotherapy thepogp.co.uk

Returning to running thepostnatalplan. com/p/returning-to-running-postpartum-with-emma-jeffery-pt

Resources for birthing injuries:

The MASIC Foundation masic.org.uk

Royal College of Obstetricians and Gynaecologists (see page 'Perineal tears during childbirth') rcog.org.uk/ for-the-public/perineal-tears-and-episiotomies-in-childbirth/perineal-tears-during-childbirth

Resources for C-section recovery:

HLP Therapy (see page 'C-Section Scar Massage') hlp-therapy. co.uk/c-section-scar-massage

HLP Therapy and Positive C-Section – Hannah Poulton youtube.com/@ ScarRecoveryHLPTherapy

Resources for pelvic organ prolapse and urinary incontinence:

National Institute for Health and Care Excellence (see page 'Urinary incontinence and pelvic organ prolapse in women: management') nice.org.uk/guidance/ng123

NHS (see page 'Non-surgical treatment: Urinary incontinence') nhs.uk/ conditions/urinary-incontinence/ treatment

Squeezy squeezyapp.com

Resources for postnatal checks:

The Mummy MOT themummymot.com

TEEN MOTHERHOOD ADVICE AND SUPPORT

PANDAS pandasfoundation.org.uk or call 0808 1961 776

Samaritans samaritans.org or call 116 123

Shout giveusashout.org or text 'YM' to 85258

WORKPLACE RIGHTS

Acas acas.org.uk

Citizens Advice citizensadvice.org.uk

GOV.UK (see page 'Pregnant employees' rights') gov.uk/working-when-pregnant-your-rights

Maternity Action maternityaction.org.uk

EXPERT BIOGRAPHIES

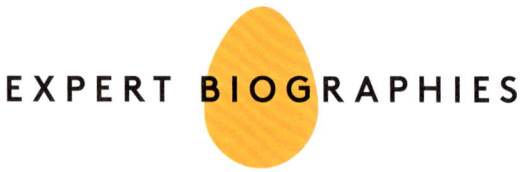

Dr Federica Amati

Dr Federica Amati holds a PhD in Clinical Medicine Research from Imperial College London, has a masters in Public Health and is an Association for Nutrition (AfN) Registered Nutritionist. She is the Nutrition Topic Lead at Imperial College London School of Medicine and is the Head Nutritionist for science and nutrition company, ZOE.

Dr Fede's approach focuses on improving overall dietary quality following the principles of evidence-based, personalised nutrition science for improved health span and disease prevention throughout the lifecourse.

Alongside her research and nutrition work, Federica has written two books, *Recipes for a Better Menopause* and Sunday Times bestseller *Every Body Should Know This*.

Website: federicaamati.com
Instagram: @dr.fede.amati

Emilie Bellet

Emilie Bellet is the founder and CEO of Vestpod.com, a community that helps people improve their financial lives through courses, events, festival, and The Wallet podcast. She is the author of *You're Not Broke, You're Pre-Rich*, which teaches you how to master your money and accomplish your financial

objectives. Emilie has a background in private equity and is a personal finance expert whose articles have been featured in media outlets like the *Financial Times* and *Vogue*.

Website: vestpod.com/
Instagram: @vestpod

Dr Caroline Boyd

Chartered clinical psychologist Dr Caroline Boyd has over 10 years' experience working in the NHS and mental health settings, and she supports parents from pregnancy to childbirth and beyond. Caroline is the author of *Mindful New Mum: A Mind-Body Approach to the Highs and Lows of Motherhood*, and her published research explores mothers' experiences of intrusive thoughts about their babies. Her work has been featured in *You* magazine, *Grazia*, and Woman's Hour on BBC Radio 4, and she is an Ambassador for UK perinatal mental health charity, PANDAS.

Caroline specialises in supporting parents around anger and anxiety in her independent psychology practice, Parent Therapy Hub. She shares psychology ideas on Instagram and in the media to help parents feel more connected – to themselves and their children – and less alone.

Website: drcarolineboyd.com
Instagram: @_drboyd

Tessa Clemson

Tessa Clemson is a specialist in pregnancy and postnatal yoga, the author of *Yogi Baby*, the host of the 'You and Your Yogi Baby' podcast, and the founder of the Tessa Clemson Yoga Studio & Wellness Space, a community hub for thousands of families.

Tessa appeared on Davina McCall's Channel 4 documentary *Pill Revolution* and her podcast 'Making the Cut', where they bonded over a shared passion for birth, supporting women and the importance of sharing positive birth experiences to inspire and educate.

As a Maternity Voices Partnership Champion, she helps review and contribute to the development and improvement of local maternity and neonatal care through service-user feedback and support.

Website: Tessaclemsonyoga.com
Instagram @tessaclemsonyoga

Five X More

The UK's leading women's health organisation focuses on Black maternal health. Their mission is to empower, support and advocate for Black women, ensuring they receive the respectful, equitable, and high-quality care they deserve during pregnancy and beyond.

Website: fivexmore.org
Instagram: @fivexmore_

Caroline Flint RN RM ADM

Caroline was inspired to become a midwife following the birth of her sister at home when she was eight years old. She has now been a midwife for nearly 50 years working in hospitals and women's homes, and was an NCT Antenatal Teacher for 47 years. Caroline has been a government advisor, and set up one of the first Birth Centres in the UK, and was formerly President of the Royal College of Midwives. Caroline has three children of her own and 12 grandchildren – nine of which she delivered. She continues to run antenatal courses for the NCT.

Caroline is the author of *Sensitive Midwifery* and *DO Birth*.

Website: carolineflintmidwife.com

Jenny Gillespie MCSP HCPC Specialist Pelvic Health Physiotherapist

Jenny Gillespie has been a chartered physiotherapist for 25 years. Initially specialising in the musculoskeletal field, she has worked in the NHS and in private practice in the UK and the Middle East. Following the birth of her three teenage children, Jenny developed a passion for postnatal and pelvic floor rehabilitation, which led her to specialise in pelvic health physiotherapy.

She is the director of The Mummy Hub Physiotherapy based in Tunbridge Wells, Kent, and also works as a pelvic health physiotherapist for Maidstone and Tunbridge Wells NHS Trust.

Jenny is a member of the POGP (Pelvic, Obstetric and Gynaecological Physiotherapy) and has completed comprehensive postgraduate training with them and many other well-respected education providers. She is a certified Mummy MOT practitioner and a qualified Pilates instructor.

Jenny is honoured to contribute to *Birthing* as she is passionate about supporting women to remain well and active through pregnancy and recover and rehabilitate effectively following birth.

Website: themummyhub.com
Instagram: @ the_mummy_hubtw

Dr Karen Gurney

Dr Karen Gurney is a consultant clinical psychologist and psychosexologist for the NHS and The Havelock Clinic, an independent sexual problems service based in London. She is the author of *Mind the Gap: The truth about desire and how to futureproof your sex life* and *How Not to Let Having Kids Ruin Your Sex Life* (Headline Home). Dr Gurney has given two TED talks and is on Instagram as @thesexdoctor.

Instagram: @thesexdoctor

IVF Babble

Tracey Bambrough, co-founder of IVFbabble and co-creator of World Fertility Day, has made remarkable contributions to supporting individuals and couples facing fertility challenges. Alongside co-founder Sara Marshall-Page, Tracey has become a prominent figure in the trying-to-conceive (TTC) community through their platform, IVFbabble.com. Together, they provide essential resources, information and encouragement to those navigating the complexities of fertility.

With an unwavering commitment to raising awareness and advocating for the TTC community, Tracey has established herself as a vital voice for fertility awareness and emotional wellbeing. Her dedication continues to inspire and empower countless individuals as they pursue their personal paths to parenthood.

IVFBabble.com
@ivfbabble

Emma Jeffery

Emma Jeffery is a specialist postnatal movement coach and founder of the multi-physio recommended online programmes The First Six Weeks and The Postnatal Plan. Emma takes a pioneering approach to help mums like you, keep yourself at the forefront, rehabilitate and get stronger after the birth of your babies. Emma gives the much needed clarity, support and programming that mums deserve around postnatal exercise and pelvic health from day one. Leaking, prolapse, abdominal separation, are not barriers to returning to exercise and Emma wants every mum to know this. Emma is on a mission to raise awareness, normalise and bust taboos around pelvic health and help mums understand the importance of strength training for life!

Website: emmajefferypt.com/
Instagram: @emmajefferypt

Emma Mills

Emma Mills is a specialist birth trauma midwife with a successful private practice; Emma also works clinically in the NHS. With 25 years' experience in midwifery, in the UK and abroad, Emma specialises in supporting anyone who has suffered a traumatic experience in their journey to becoming a parent. Her unique expertise, knowledge and skills in this area came about through her recognition for the need to support and offer recovery form the hugely debilitating symptoms of birth trauma, often impacting the whole family for years after.

'You may not have had the perfect birth but with the right support you will be able to look back without fear, anxiety and panic. You are able to move forward and enjoy family life symptom free.'

Website: emmamillsmidwife.com
Instagram: @birth_therapy

Dr Louise Oliver

Dr Louise Oliver is a GP with an interest in women's health, a functional breathing practitioner and therapeutic life coach. She became a perimenopausal snorer, which led her to recognise her 24-hour breathing was inefficient. She improved her breathing efficiency, her snoring stopped, her sleep, exercise tolerance and stress resilience improved. Louise is raising awareness about how the hormonal changes occurring at puberty, pregnancy and menopause may negatively impact breathing, and encouraging those affected to change how they breathe. She now splits her time between working as a GP and functional breathing practitioner, teaching others to breathe efficiently on her individual and group breathing re-education programmes.

Website: drlouiseolivertherapeutic lifecoaching.com/
Instagram @drlouiseolivertlc

ACKNOWLEDGEMENTS

I'd like to thank my children. Every day you teach me something new. You make me laugh, you make me proud and you make me want to be a better person. Thank you for everything. Michael, there's not enough space here for what I want to say, but I think you know.

Caroline Flint, thank you for blowing everything I thought about childbirth out of the water. Ten days' bed rest changed my life. Mandy, Greg, Immie, Devon, Clemmie and Pearce – you made me a better mum.

A huge thank you to everybody at HQ for your support and belief in this book, especially Danielle Pender, Louise McKeever and Lisa Milton, and Imogen Fortes, for your patience and brilliance. I'd like to thank Amanda Harris and my agents at YMU. I love you guys. Thank you to Jonathan Hackford especially, for your patience with all my mad ideas.

Thank you to Imagist, for the beautiful design. The look and feel of this book was paramount to me and you've captured it so brilliantly.

A big thank you to Marley Henry for sharing all your wisdom and knowledge. The book needed your practical advice and calm reassurance and I am so grateful to have found you. And thank you to all our contributors, such a talented group of experts who have offered their advice and guidance so generously: Dr Federica Amati, Emilie Bellet, Dr Caroline Boyd, Tessa Clemson, Clo and Tinuke – founders of Five X More,

Jenny Gillespie, Dr Karen Gurney, Emma Jeffery, Emma Mills and Dr Louise Oliver and Sara Marshall-Page and Tracey Bambrough and Harry Baker for his amazing poem, Trying. Big shout-out to all the midwives out there. You are amazing. And to the obstetricians whom we often only get to see during labour in an emergency.

I particularly want to say thank you to all the beautiful women and partners who have shared their birthing stories. Many of them were great experiences but some of them were very difficult and I just wanted you to know how I grateful I am to you all for opening up and giving your experiences to others. Everyone reading this book will get so much from them, so thank you from the bottom of my heart.

FROM MARLEY:

Thanks to my biggest cheerleader, Tyrone, my husband. Thank you for always being there. I also wouldn't be where I am now without my mum Lorraine guiding, teaching and supporting me all these years. My children, all 5 of them, have given me so much joy, and experience. I love you all.

Thank you to all the parents who have let me be a part of your birth experience and early parenthood journey. Lastly, a HUGE thank you to Davina (she is the best!) and HQ for inviting me to be a part of this masterpiece, which I know will serve expectant parents everywhere, helping them to have a better birth.

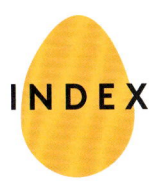

INDEX

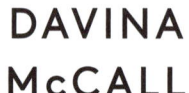

DAVINA McCALL

Davina McCall is a well-loved television personality and is best known for presenting *Big Brother*, *The Masked Singer* and *My Mum, Your Dad*.

Davina is a passionate advocate and champion for women's health issues and has made several documentaries on the subject: *Pill Revolution*; *Let's Talk Sex*; *Sex, Myths and the Menopause*; and *Sex, Mind and the Menopause*.

As a mother of three, she passionately believes that every woman's access to care during pregnancy and childbirth must be guaranteed, ensuring they can experience birth in the way they truly desire and deserve.

@davinamccall